Praise for *Real Words with Sam*

J Brad Britton taught me one of the most important principles that shaped my life and work: *Do the right thing, not the easy thing.* In *Real Words with Sam*, J Brad reveals how he had to relearn this lesson in the most humbling way possible - from his own son.

The heart of this book isn't about autism or alternative communication methods, though you'll learn about both. It's about what happens when we finally stop trying to fix people and start listening to them. J Brad's journey from presuming incompetence to presuming competence with Sam will challenge how you see everyone in your life.

Real Words with Sam is honest, uncomfortable at times, and ultimately transformative. If you've ever underestimated someone - or been underestimated yourself - this story will stay with you long after you finish reading."

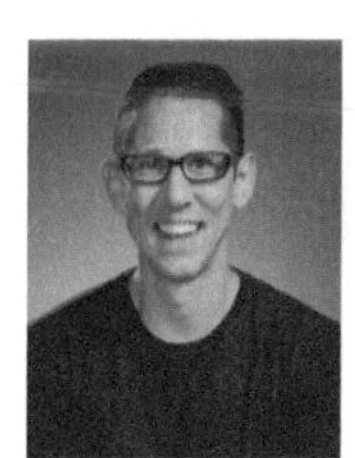

~ Hal Elrod,
bestselling author of 12 books, including
The Miracle Morning and
The Miracle Equation

In two decades as an autism educator, parent, and through co-founding Spellers Method, I've learned that presuming competence isn't just good practice—it's a moral imperative. *Real Words with Sam* makes that truth undeniable. J Brad Britton bares his soul as a humble father who deeply loves his son but misunderstood him for decades. He lays bare the divide between Sam's actual intelligence and what others saw, and demonstrates how spelling connected them. The book's format—alternating between father's reflection and Sam's own spelled thoughts—challenges every reader to examine their assumptions. This is truly a transformative read for anyone who works with or loves someone who communicates differently!

~ Dawnmarie Gaivin, Spellers Method Co-creator / Exec Director of Spellers Freedom Foundation

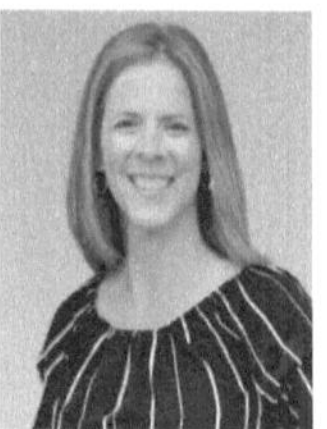

I've long respected J. Brad Britton as a leader. But in *Real Words with Sam*, he models the rarest kind of leadership—the courage to confront his own assumptions.

This book is not just about autism. It's about awakening. It's about a father who had the humility to confront his own assumptions and the courage to truly listen. The story will challenge you to presume competence, look beyond appearances, and believe there is always more beneath the surface.

The real Sam is revealed in these pages. And if you allow it, Sam's story can also reveal a newer, better version of you.

~ Dan Casetta

Real Words With Sam: A Father and Son Navigate Autism, Apraxia, and Unexpected Intelligence by J Brad and Sam Britton challenges every assumption we make about intelligence when someone's body won't cooperate with their mind. This book delivers what most autism stories don't. Sam's actual voice, spelled out letter by letter, proving his intelligence was there all along while the world assumed otherwise. J Brad's story of discovering he'd been having a one-sided conversation with his son for twenty years is both heart-activating, eye-opening, and transformative (whether you have a child with, or know someone with autism, or not!).

What hit me most was J Brad's framework of presuming understanding versus misunderstanding. I see this play out constantly with misaligned leaders who overlook the intelligence in their teams simply because it doesn't show up in expected ways. J Brad's deep vulnerability about underestimating Sam for years and the complete mindset reset required to truly see his son forced ME to examine where I might be doing the same thing in my own life. This is the kind of book that shifts how you see people and the world at large, period.

If you've ever worked with, loved, or wanted to understand someone who communicates differently, this book is absolutely a must-read!!

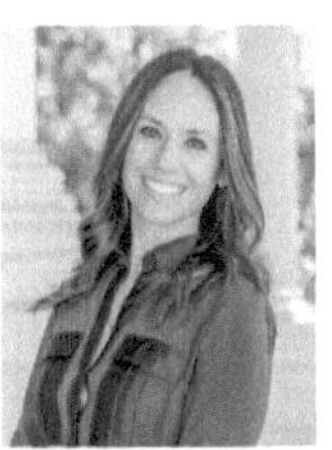

~ Amber Vilhauer
Books & Business Strategist,
#1 Bestselling Author,
Inc5000 CEO, NGNG Enterprises

———

Real Words with Sam offers a raw and moving look at communication, autonomy, and the impact of our beliefs about people who have unreliable speech. Through Sam's voice and his dad's reflections, this book challenges deficit-based narratives and replaces them with curiosity, respect, and possibility.

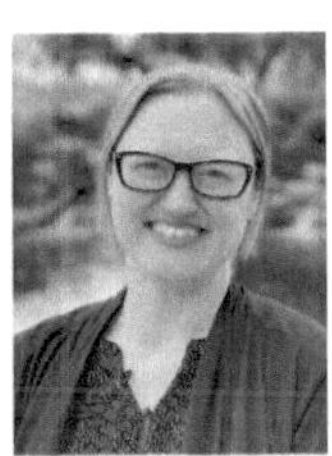

~ Julie Sando,
Co-Director of Communication
For Education / Director of Autistically
Inclined

Real Words with Sam is a powerful book about seeing the people you love more clearly and learning to recognize who they're becoming every day.

J Brad's journey with Sam is honest, humbling, and real. It's about challenging your own assumptions, growing as a parent, and learning to truly listen. As a father, this struck a chord and got me thinking about how I show up for my own daughter.

I've always believed family and relationships come first. But without intentional growth, those words can become empty. This book is a reminder that being the parent our kids need takes humility and self-awareness.

Sam's voice will change how you think about communication, intelligence, and what's possible.

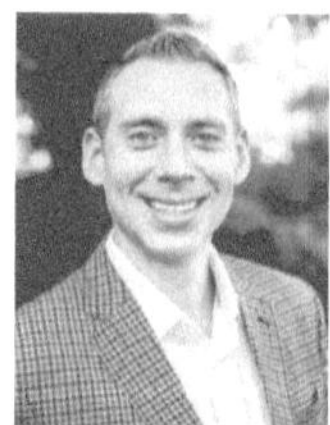

~ **Justin Donald,**
#1 WSJ and USA Today Best-Selling Author of *The Lifestyle Investor*, Founder of The Lifestyle Investor Mastermind, Host of The Lifestyle Investor Podcast

Real Words
with S A M

Real Words
with S A M

a father and son navigate autism,
apraxia, and unexpected intelligence

J BRAD AND SAM BRITTON

Visit the author's website at: www.RealWordsWithSam.com/resources

Published and distributed by: STRONGPrint Publishing

Real Words With Sam: A Father and Son Navigate Autism, Apraxia, and Unexpected Intelligence

ISBN: 978-1-962074-31-5 Hardcover
ISBN: 978-1-962074-29-2 Paperback
ISBN: 978-1-962074-30-8 ebook

Dedicated to the underestimated and misunderstood

Contents

Introduction
Before We Get Started

I had no idea I'd been having a one-sided conversation with my son for two decades.

I've spent my life valuing clear communication.

And yet . . . I missed it.

Not because I wasn't trying. Not because I didn't care. But because I didn't know what I didn't know.

Looking back, it's humbling. I'd have put myself near the bottom of the list of people likely to overlook something so vital. But that's the thing about perspective. One shift, one new piece of understanding, can be like stepping into a new world.

This book is about my shift. About discovering my son had been listening, understanding, and thinking deeply all along. While I mostly just saw disability.

I'm an autism parent.

An autism dad.

That means I'm raising a child on the autism spectrum and learning to see through a different lens.

If you're reading this, chances are you care about someone on the autism spectrum and want to understand and support them better. You might be a parent, a sibling, a friend, or a teacher. Maybe you're not even sure what brought you here.

That's okay. There's something here for you.

So what is this, really? A guide? A confession? A lifeline?

It's stories. Real stories. Raw, personal moments that usually stay tucked away.

Whether you're walking a similar path or trying to understand someone who is, these pages offer something: practical wisdom for parents, guidance for supporters, and for everyone, a glimpse into how assumptions can evolve and relationships can deepen with new awareness.

Think of this as a map, but not the kind with a direct route from point A to point B. It's the kind marked with detours that turned out to be destinations. Imagine notes scribbled in the margins about things discovered along the way:

"Pause here for beauty."

"This detour was worth it."

"Here be dragons…and grace."

The early miles might feel steep. There are some hard truths I need to cover first, foundations that help everything else make sense. But the terrain evens out. There are plenty of moments of joy, humor, and simple connection ahead.

Autism is not one thing. As the saying goes, *"If you've met one person with autism, you've met one person with autism."* So maybe this book isn't just one thing either: part story, part guide, part invitation to walk a stretch of the road with me. And Sam. My son.

If something in these pages helps you understand a family member, a friend, or even yourself a little better—if it brings more clarity or encouragement—I'll be grateful.

This is just one family's truth. Not a blueprint, not a definition, but an invitation to take this detour with us.

Chapter 1
I Didn't Want To

On September 26, 2024, I decided to write this book, and unexpectedly found myself crying. That surprise hit me hard, urging me to understand why.

I didn't want to write it. I still don't, not really. There's a big part of me that wants to avoid it altogether. Writing it means reliving things I've kept inside for years. It means unpacking feelings that I usually manage by moving forward, rather than dwelling on them.

But something in me knows I need to write it. Maybe it's for Sam—to make sure his story is fully seen and heard. Maybe it's for other families walking a similar path. Perhaps it's for people who have never thought much about autism but want to gain a deeper understanding. Or maybe it's just for me to face what I've carried, cast a light, and see what's really there.

I believe each reader will take away something uniquely their own.

I'm not someone who usually shows strong feelings, especially the kind that bring tears.

Enthusiasm, optimism, gratitude? Easy for me.

Regret, frustration, or despair? I tend to keep those to myself.

That's why the tears caught me off guard. I realized this would demand a level of openness I rarely allow—a vulnerability I'd need to embrace to share my story as Sam's dad honestly. If I want it to matter, I'll have to step past my usual stoicism and share the parts I've kept hidden: the helplessness, the doubt, the fear.

That moment of tears wasn't just about me. I know I'm not alone in that. Many men are taught to keep their deepest struggles private. Not because we don't feel them, but because we're unsure how or when to share them. And for those who don't relate, I hope this offers a window into the world of men like me, who find it easier to stay silent than to speak the truth of what we're carrying.

For me, that tendency toward silence often shows up as composure. I've always taken pride in staying emotionally steady, rarely too high or too low. It's how I was raised, and how I've grown to function.

This steadiness is part of emotional intelligence, or EQ, which involves managing our reactions when things become challenging. One common explanation puts it this way:

"A cornerstone of EQ is the ability to manage one's reactions. People with low EQ may struggle to control their emotions and might have unexpected emotional outbursts."

For most of my life, I've lived by a simple mantra: "Can't change it."

It's been my way of navigating life's challenges by focusing on what I can control and letting go of what I can't. That mindset has served me well in my work, my relationships, and most of all, in the journey of being an autism dad, where I've learned to release what I can't control and hold tight to what I can.

As I dig into what this process is revealing, I realize it's not always that simple.

When *can't change it* falls short, faith anchors and helps me trust there's a purpose, even in uncertainty. Love may push us forward, but faith keeps us grounded.

When it comes to my son, Sam, the stoic *can't change it* philosophy helps me navigate challenges. It doesn't address the deeper emotions, though. The anxiety. The frustration. The helplessness.

Writing is making me face it. The more I dig, the more I realize it's hidden feelings, ones I've rarely voiced, that have shaped my path the most.

As Sam's dad, I've learned to see my feelings through a simple lens: love and fear. Love drives my joy and hope; fear fuels my anxiety and doubts. That perspective helps me navigate the challenges of parenting him.

My wife, Paulette, is an autism mom. She's deeply connected to the autism community. She knows countless people across the country (and even internationally) who find support and strength there. Through her, I've glimpsed that world, but I haven't been very active in it. In twenty years, I've been to fewer than a dozen autism-related events, and frankly, only one stands out as truly valuable. I'll share that story soon, along with a few more about the amazing woman I married.

And then there's Sam's older sister, Madison. Just as Paulette is our link to the autism community, Madison is the one who keeps it real at home. She doesn't take any flak from Sam, never has, and she doesn't give him much slack either. She's his biggest protector, but also his fiercest challenger. She'll fight for him in a heartbeat, and just as quickly tell him when he's out of line.

Their relationship isn't perfect, but it's authentic. She picks on him. He annoys her.

Yet beneath it all is a bond built on love, loyalty, and mutual respect. And maybe most importantly, she treats him like a little brother, not a diagnosis. And because of that, Sam listens to her. He works hard for her approval. He knows she sees him, and that means more than words can say.

The tears that surprised me that day weren't really about writing a book. They were about Sam. He's 24 years old now, and still teaching me every day.

Sam has transformed my life in ways I couldn't have imagined.

My bond with him runs deep, and I've come to respect him at a level that I believe only an autism parent can fully understand. Watching Sam grow has been a privilege. Moreover, his growth has encouraged me to grow as well.

Recently, at church, the pastor quoted best-selling author Erwin McManus:

"If your purpose is rooted in success, your purpose is fragile.

But if your purpose is rooted in the person you become, it is untouchable."

It's a truth I've believed for years.

Easy to repeat.

Harder to live.

Especially for those of us who measure success in careers, achievements, or outcomes, that quote hits differently. I've shared it with others. Living it takes work. Success can fade, but who we become endures.

While I hope you'll find ideas, tips, and maybe even strategies to help you face hard things, that's not my purpose.

My purpose is to share a relatable experience. Everyone faces challenges. They may look different, but underneath, the feelings are often the same.

Through my relationship with Sam, I've discovered insights I believe can resonate with anyone going through hard things.

There have been times when no amount of reasoning or problem-solving could bring comfort. In those moments, when nothing made sense, faith didn't solve the problem— but it steadied me enough to keep believing that something greater was at work.

Some of the strongest people I know are friends who have faced unimaginable hardships with optimism, grace, and belief. They helped me realize that growth comes from facing fear, not avoiding it.[1]

Writing this book will require vulnerability. I'll talk about feeling lost, underestimating Sam, and doubting myself as a father. But I'll also share the immense love, joy, and gratitude that come from being Sam's dad.

This story isn't just for autism families.

It's for anyone who has faced the fear of the unknown or the doubt of not being enough. Parenting Sam has shown me that while the specifics of our challenges differ, the emotions we face, love and fear, are universal.

The hardest moments come when I confront my limitations as Sam's dad. When he's struggling and I can't find the cause fast enough, when I fail to prevent a meltdown,

---

[1]   I think especially of two men I deeply admire: Hal Elrod and Bruce Goodman. Both have faced life-threatening battles with leukemia and walked through them with extraordinary courage, faith, and grit. Their stories and their ongoing impact on my life helped shape my story more than they know.

when I sit there wondering if I'm doing enough for him, it's overwhelming.

But this uncertainty isn't unique to autism parenting.

It's part of being a parent. It's part of being human.

Love sustains me, especially when I doubt myself as Sam's dad, or can't ease his struggles. It's the bond I share with Sam, the simple and profound affection that steadies me. And when love alone can't carry me forward, faith steps in. Together, they build resilience: the quiet strength to keep going, one step at a time.

Introduction Continued
More Things You Should Know

(A chapter that's not a chapter)

Who is Sam Britton?

My son.

24 years old and I'm still discovering the full depth of who he is.

I hope this book helps uncover that, not just for you, but for me.

Reflecting on our experiences and putting them into written form deepens my comprehension of who Sam is and how our relationship continues to grow. And before we go further, there are a few essential things to share, pieces of background that will help the rest of the chapters make more sense.

These truths will unfold through our stories, especially in Sam's own words. But some things are worth saying up front.

The stories here weave together moments from across two decades and don't follow a strict timeline. Some look back to Sam's early years, others reflect on more recent experiences. This isn't Sam's story told in chronological order. It's our relationship explored through the moments that shaped us most.

Let me start here:

Sam does not have a learning disability.

That might surprise people, especially those who meet him for the first time or spend only a few minutes with him. His body moves in ways that may seem unusual. His words don't always match the moment. At first glance, it's easy to assume there's a cognitive delay or intellectual disability.

But that assumption is wrong.

Sam's challenge isn't comprehension. It's expression.

He doesn't have trouble taking in information. He has trouble getting it out.

This disconnect has a name: apraxia.

It's a motor planning disorder.

When a person can say a few words but can't hold a conversation (or quotes entire scenes from YouTube, but struggles answering yes/no questions), it's tempting to assume there's a learning disorder.

That's why so many people with autism are misunderstood. Their spoken words—or the absence of them—don't reflect the intelligence, insight, or emotional depth that's really there.

It's not a speech problem. It's a movement problem.

It's why someone like Sam can spell a profound insight or a poetic turn of phrase, yet still be unable to answer a simple verbal question on cue.

That's apraxia.

And once you understand it, things start to look different.

It's not a language delay.

It's not a behavioral quirk.

And it's certainly not a lack of intelligence.

It doesn't just affect speech. It can affect anything that requires voluntary movement. For Sam, apraxia can make even simple tasks take enormous effort. Walking from here to there, following instructions, initiating movement, or stopping a repetitive behavior can all become uphill battles. His brain is firing clear commands, but his body misfires or freezes.

Sometimes, the signal gets through.

Sometimes, it doesn't.

And sometimes, the harder he tries, the worse it gets.

In *The Speller's Guidebook*, authors Dawnmarie Gaivin and Dana Johnson describe apraxia this way:

"Apraxia is a disconnect between intention and initiation. The mind knows what it wants to do. The body doesn't always cooperate."

That one line explains more about my son's experience than years of therapy reports ever could.

Here's something that might surprise you: According to a 2015 PubMed study, apraxia affects roughly 67% of people diagnosed with autism. Think about that for a moment. Two-thirds of people with autism may be experiencing this same disconnect between mind and body. That statistic can completely reframe how we see and hear those who struggle to communicate.

Apraxia doesn't always show itself clearly. From the outside, it might look like stubbornness. Or inattention. Or disobedience.

You might see it in something called echolalia: when a person repeats words, phrases, or sounds they've heard before, often from TV shows, songs, or people around them.

You might also see it in something called stimming (short for self-stimulatory behavior). Repetitive movements or sounds that help regulate emotion or sensory input. It might look like flapping hands, bouncing, or rocking. Some kids wave objects like straws or pens in front of their eyes to watch the motion. Others pace, spin, hum, or clap.

To an outsider, echolalia and stimming may seem random or out of place, but for the person with apraxia, it's a way of processing language, self-soothing, or communicating indirectly.

But on the inside?

It can feel like being locked out of the body. Fully aware, yet unable to respond in the way you want.

And that must be more frustrating for them than for anyone else.

Even when Sam uses his own words instead of repeating others, apraxia still interferes. That's what makes him what's known as an unreliable speaker.

He can say words, but often, those words aren't what he means. Sometimes they are. Sometimes they aren't. That inconsistency is what makes them unreliable.

His voice isn't always under his control. Not the words, not the timing, and definitely not the volume. And because of that, we've learned not to judge his intelligence by what comes out of his mouth.

That makes understanding him a daily challenge—and sometimes, a daily heartbreak.

His speech doesn't always reflect his thoughts.

But spelling does.

Sam spells his thoughts one letter at a time using a simple letterboard with a communication partner's support.

It's a process that takes patience, effort, and years of practice. And it's still unfolding.

Since Sam began spelling, much has changed, not only in how he communicates but also in how I see him and understand his mind. In just four years, that comprehension has grown more than it did in twenty years before.

He's revealing himself in unexpected ways.

I use the word "unexpected" intentionally.

When asked, "What is something you find rewarding?" Sam spelled:

ALL THE TIMES THAT I ASTOUND
OTHER PEOPLE WITH MY UNEXPECTED
INTELLIGENCE.

I know, right?

My respect for his mind and his resilience has grown exponentially.

I used to think I knew him well. Now, I know better: I'm still learning who he is, one letter at a time.

What matters is this:

Spelling is giving Sam
a more reliable voice.

And you'll hear it throughout.

You may have noticed Sam is listed as a **co-author.**

That's not a gesture. It's the truth.

Yes, this book is about my experiences as Sam's dad, but it's also about his experiences.

And many of the most powerful words are his.

You'll find them in the pages titled **Real Words** *with* **Sam.**

Each time, you'll be reading real words spelled by Sam.

Sometimes as direct answers to questions, and sometimes as spontaneous thoughts that emerged during sessions.

Words spelled letter by letter, in moments built on trust, perseverance, and deliberate effort.

Nothing has been rewritten or polished. You're seeing exactly what he shared with us.

Where helpful, I've added brief notes for context.

These aren't imagined dialogues or polished essays.

They're glimpses into Sam's heart and mind, exactly as he chose to express them.

More than words.

They're his voice, finding its way into the world.

And to us, that's priceless.

Finally, one more thing you'll probably notice:

Sam's writing has a distinct rhythm: poetic, lyrical, sometimes formal, sometimes surprising.

While I can't replicate Sam's voice, I've leaned into a similar rhythm. One that values flow over grammar, cadence over convention.

I hope that choice helps you feel what this is about, not just intellectually, but emotionally.

Because these aren't just stories. They're glimpses into a relationship that's still growing, into a life that's always been richer than it appeared, into a young man who's been thinking profound thoughts and waiting—for years, even decades—for a way to share them.

And now, finally, he can.

Real Words *with* Sam

Tell me one word you think of when you hear the word snail?

SLIME

What do you think about the idea of eating Sakondry bugs?

THE IDEA IS GOOD TO SAVE THE LEMURS
BUT NOT FOR ME

What is one thing civilizations might rival over?

LAND THE RULERS WANT TO BUILD
THEIR LAND ON

Summarize in your own words why Alexander Selkirk was
left on a remote island?

ITS ALL BECAUSE GUYS ARE TOO
HOT TEMPERED

AND HE GOT INTO A DISPUTE WITH
THE CAPTAIN

What do you think is meant by the phrase humble
circumstances?

TO START WITH LITTLE
MATERIALISTIC THINGS

What do you want to say to your dad?

TO THE BEST DAD FOR ME

I VERY MUCH WANT YOU TO KNOW THAT I
LOVE YOU

TIME ONLY CONTINUES TO BUILD OUR BOND

Chapter 2
Hidden in Plain Sight

I walked into the symposium half-skeptical, half-supportive. We'd tried so many things already, and I wasn't expecting much. Certainly not to have my assumptions shattered in under three minutes.

It was 2018, and my wife, Paulette, had told me about the event a few weeks earlier.

The subject was Spelled Communication, an approach that helps non-speakers share their thoughts using letter-boards and keyboards.

Over the years, we saw many therapies come and go. Some seemed to help a little. Some barely at all. What worked wonders for one child often had little to no effect on another.

As mentioned in the introduction, there's a saying in the autism community: *"If you've met one person with autism, you've met one person with autism."* Sam had already taught us that, in a way only he could.

And maybe, without realizing it, I had grown a little callous toward new ideas. Perhaps I had become a little too good at managing my expectations.

That's probably why I walked into the symposium feeling cautious, maybe even skeptical.

I hadn't done any real research. I hadn't seen it in action. But I agreed to go.

We drove a few hours to the college campus hosting the event. We joined a crowd of about 150 people walking toward the main building.

As we walked into one of the main gathering rooms, where the presentations would take place, we saw a woman named Julie standing with Elliot.

Julie is a spelling coach. I'm not sure if that's her official title, but it fits.

As we approached, Julie turned to Elliot and said, "Hey, I think you recognize these people," gesturing toward Paulette and me.

Paulette immediately replied, "Oh, yes! We've met a few times. He's from our hometown of Fallbrook and the same age as Sam."

I realized that I had met him before, eight or ten years earlier, when he was about seven years old.

At the time, he was energetic—bouncing on his toes, flapping his hands, repeating random words and sounds with an infectious smile.

Now, at around 15 years old, he still had the same vibrant energy.

As he bounced, making excited sounds—"eeee!"—Julie held up a laminated letterboard in front of him.

About 12 by 9 inches. Simple, nothing fancy. One side had the alphabet, the other, numbers and punctuation.

Julie asked if he wanted to say hello.

And then we watched something extraordinary.

Still bouncing and flapping, he began poking letters on the board slowly, painstakingly, one at a time.

As he touched the board, Julie called out each letter, so we could follow along.

It took about two minutes, and this is what he spelled:

"Hello, fellow Fallbrookians. How are the life and times of Sam Britton these days?"

I got chills.

Tears formed in my eyes, and my jaw dropped.

That thoughtful, articulate sentence had been inside his mind all along.

In that instant, my feelings toward him changed. Not because I suddenly "respected" him (I like to believe I've always respected people as a baseline), but because I realized how much I had underestimated him. I had seen the bouncing, the flapping, the loudness . . . but not the brilliant mind fighting to be heard.

I had known him for years, in a way.

But that day, I met him for the first time.

And almost just as quickly, the possibilities for Sam began rushing into focus.

It was inspiring, but I didn't immediately assume Sam could do the same.

Hope was there, quiet and cautious.

Still, it was hope.

Throughout the symposium, we heard from dozens of spelling coaches, teachers, and parents.

We saw videos of non- speakers who, as children, exhibited the same kinds of behaviors we knew well. Loudness, echolalia, meltdowns, stimming.

We learned something critical: Much of what looked like 'behavior problems' was actually apraxia—minds trapped by bodies that wouldn't cooperate.

And right there in front of us, these same people we'd seen in videos showed us that they were far more than a diagnosis or a list of behaviors. It was staggering. Using keyboards, letterboards, or iPads, they told stories that were intelligent, aware, and eloquent. Even thinking back on it now, my head shakes back and forth in amazement.

By the time we left the symposium, we knew one thing for sure:

We had to give Sam this chance.

We left with a cautious hope and a plan. Sam would start spelling. It was time to listen.

Real Words *with* Sam

What animal language would you study?

> GIRAFFE

Why?

> THOSE GIRAFFES LISTEN TO EVERYONE

What might make a cow happy?

> NOT ROTTEN FOOD

Name a negative emotion?

> LONELY

What might make a cow sad?

> PULLING TOO HARD ON ITS UDDERS

What do you think could have been a problem with having real life animals in this original ride at Disney?

> THEY POOP EVERYWHERE

Chapter 3
Presume Competence

At first, I thought the symposium changed how I saw the boy with the letterboard. But soon, I realized it changed how I saw my own son.

Among families like ours, one phrase echoes louder than most, simple and life-changing:

Non-speaking isn't non-thinking.

It didn't happen all at once, but over time, this understanding exposed something I hadn't realized about myself.

Without meaning to, I had spent years assuming that if someone couldn't speak clearly, they couldn't think clearly either.

I never would've said it out loud.

I don't think I would have even admitted it to myself.

But looking back, I can see it now, in the way I talked about Sam when he was standing right beside me, as if he couldn't understand.

In the way I apologized for him in public, assuming he couldn't process what was happening around him.

In the way I lowered my expectations without even noticing it.

There's a brutal kind of honesty in facing that truth.

It's not that I didn't love Sam. Of course I did.

It's not that I didn't respect him. I believed I did.

But in one critical way, I'd failed:

I hadn't presumed competence.

Two words. Presume competence. Simple to say. Much harder to live.

Because presuming competence meant admitting I hadn't been doing it.

I hadn't treated Sam like someone with a mind full of brilliant thoughts, wise insights, and rich feelings.

Believing in someone's intelligence doesn't make communication easy overnight. It just stops you from underestimating what's already there.

Seeing a non-speaker spell for the first time didn't erase all my old habits. It cracked something open, but the real work was just beginning.

Slowly (painfully slowly at times) I started seeing how often I still spoke about Sam as if he weren't there.

How often I used words I never would have used with a neurotypical man his age.

How often I let old patterns slip through without thinking.

Even today, there are moments when Paulette and I catch ourselves talking about Sam, right in front of him, as if he can't hear us.

Old habits take time to unlearn.

But the more we get to know Sam, the more we presume competence, even when we don't see the evidence right away. The more we believe, the more he reveals: his intelligence, his wit, his heart.

It's not enough to love someone.

It's not enough to be patient, or kind, or good-hearted.

If we don't believe in their intelligence—if we don't presume they have something meaningful to say—we are stealing something vital from them.

Their dignity.

Their voice.

The truth we learned at the symposium: *Non-speaking isn't non-thinking.*

Once Sam had the tools he needed to spell, to type, to get his thoughts into the world, we began to see the depth that had been there all along.

What we found was more than understanding.

It was wisdom.

It was heart.

It was him.

Real Words *with* Sam

Name one thing you would find out in the jungle?

DANGER

What is one thing Tarzan is known for?

DARING ADVENTURE

Describe what you think it would be like to be raised by apes?

TO CREATE BELOVED HABITS SHAPED BY
APES WOULD TRULY BE SOMETHING UNIQUE

Why do you think this movie was so successful?

SO EASY TO LOVE A MOVIE FULL OF CATCHY
MUSIC AND COLORFUL CHARACTERS

What qualities and characteristics do you think make someone brave?

HOW SOMEONE EXHIBITS BRAVERY DEPENDS
ON THEIR OWN LIFE EXPERIENCES

IT CAN LOOK DIFFERENT ON EACH
PERSON BRAVERY COMES OUT WHEN
WE NEED IT MOST

Chapter 4
First Sam, Then Dad

Whether it's crowded or not doesn't matter. Sam loves taking a number at the barbershop. He pulls a number and waits for his turn. Even if nobody else is waiting, even if the staff isn't using the numbers that day, Sam has to pull one.

Today, we walked in, and it was one of those quiet days. No one was waiting.

Sam walked straight over and pulled a number anyway: 97.

I grabbed a number, too: 98.

Almost every time we go for haircuts, I hear the same phrase:

"First Sam, then Dad." On our walks there, I stay about five feet behind him, close enough to be present, far enough to let him lead.

It's a structure he counts on, especially on harder days. But today wasn't one of those days. Today, everything moved like clockwork.

I looked up at the digital display: 21.

It must have been a slower day, and they weren't advancing the numbers, but Sam wasn't about to get up until his number was called.

The staff knows Sam. They're kind, patient, and generous.

Without missing a beat, they clicked the remote and advanced the display to 97.

His face lit up as the number changed.

He stood tall, walked over, dropped his number in the trash can, and proudly sat down in chair number five, counting the chairs to announce his spot. *"ONE, TWO, THREE, FOUR . . . CHAIR NUMBER FIVE!"*

Everyone knew he was here!

He tends to speak about three or four notches louder than necessary, part of his natural exuberance. It takes a great deal of focus and intentionality for him to talk with "appropriate volume," and we're working on it. He's getting better.

The barber tried to put the cape around his neck.

But before she could secure it, Sam noticed something essential was missing: No one had advanced the number for me.

Sam popped up, marched to the remote control, and clicked the display forward to 98.

Order must be preserved; first Sam, then Dad.

I stood and gave Sam's barber some simple instructions.

"Regular boy's haircut. Clippers on the side at one-and-a-half. Take about a half-inch off the top. Rounded in the back."

We were good to go.

I sat down in chair number one.

Sam was three seats away, softly talking to himself, a steady stream of random phrases and cheerful words.

His volume was relatively mild. (Hallelujah, amen.)

I could barely hear him from where I sat.

The barber finished Sam's haircut, and with it came a return to full Sam volume:

"Oh, thanks so much! What a cool haircut!"

Pure, unfiltered gratitude.

Sam went to the waiting chairs to sit patiently while I finished my haircut.

I could see him out of the corner of my eye, and I noticed him stand up and start walking to the other end of the shop.

There's a restroom back there, and he's been there before, so that's where I assumed he was going.

Still, just to be sure, I asked my barber quietly,

"Can you tell where he's going?"

She glanced up, her eyes following him, a little confused at first.

Then, across the shop, came Sam's unmistakable voice, three notches above normal, per the usual:

"Biiiggg Huuggg!"

I stood up, turned, and took a step toward him.

Sure enough, there he was, hugging his barber.

It was a gentle embrace, not a tight squeeze, and, thank God, she was smiling and patting his back lightly.

I didn't want to yell across the room.

Instead, in a firm but calm voice, just loud enough to carry, I said,

"That's enough hugging. Three . . . two . . . one."

And like a charm, it worked.

Sam gently released his hug and returned to the waiting chairs.

As he sat down, Sam looked over at me.

He could tell, just from my expression, that I wasn't happy.

The hug had already happened; no changing that. But this wasn't new.

We've had plenty of conversations about when it's okay to hug and when it's not.

Sam knows the rules. He really does. But sometimes, when excitement bubbles up, his body moves faster than his mind.

Fortunately, the shop itself answered with kindness.

I heard a few good-natured oohs and aahs from around the room.

One of the other barbers laughed and said, "I'm jealous. My customers don't hug me!"

Another joked, "That's a better tip than I usually get."

Sam, picking up on my disappointment, decided to stand up, walk over to me while I was still sitting in my barber's chair, and offer me a hug. I've learned this is Sam's apology language—not words he can't reliably summon, but touch he can control. The hug says what his voice can't: "I heard you. I understand. I'm trying." Maybe it's also his way of doing a little sucking up. (He's known for that move.)

That earned another warm "Awww" from the room.

He sat back down, a perfect gentleman, while my haircut finished.

When it was time to pay, I tipped my barber generously and gave Sam money to tip his barber even more generously.

A small token of appreciation for her kindness.

Sam waved and called out cheerful goodbyes:

"Bye, everybody! See you next time!"

I smiled and offered a grateful nod.

We stepped outside, the afternoon sun on our faces, Sam marching proudly a few steps ahead.

And just like that, we were walking home—numbers pulled, haircuts done, order preserved.

Real Words *with* Sam

What topic would you like to do research on?

LIVING ON THE MOON

Do you think you could live in a satellite in space?

I THINK TO ORBIT PLANETS DOES
SEEM INCREDIBLE

What is something you would like to do this summer?

I WOULD LIKE TO EAT OUT PLAYING
ON THE BEACH

Elaborate on the "eat out by the beach" statement.

I'M THINKING THE RESTAURANT

If you could build a bridge, what two places would you
connect to each other?

IF I DESIGNED A BRIDGE NATIONAL PEOPLE IN
CALIFORNIA WOULD CONNECT TO SPACE

What do you think of skateboard clothing styles?

SKATER CLOTHES ARE NOT AS
COOL AS THEY THINK

Chapter 5
How Spelling Sessions Work
(The Technical Stuff)

This chapter is going to feel different.

More structured. More technical.

Here's what a spelling session feels like: the rhythm, the hurdles, and the moments when his voice rises to the surface.

We use the Speller's Method, a structured approach that enables Sam to communicate by spelling out words on a board, touching individual letters one at a time. It's built on a simple truth: Sam is intelligent and aware. He just needs support to share his thoughts.

Sessions typically last 50 minutes, although some days Sam may need more or less time, depending on what his body or mind is processing. This variability reminds me that his pace is part of his progress.

A session begins on Sam's terms, not with spelling or questions, but with whatever he brings into the room. Some days, Sam strides in with bright eyes, ready to begin immediately. Other days, it takes 20 minutes for him to settle into his chair. He might repeat a phrase like "Wash clothes on Friday," which seems random, but it carries weight for him. His mind might be stuck, replaying an upcoming event or a thought he can't shake, unable to move forward despite wanting to. That's when support is vital—a gentle nudge like, "Sam, you're stuck. Take a breath. You've got this." That steady encouragement helps Sam shift and focus, preparing to think and respond. In those shifts, I glimpse the voice that's been waiting.

Once Sam is settled, the coach reads a short, engaging passage from a carefully selected topic. Topics like marine biology or jazz music are chosen to spark his interest and challenge his mind.

The material is divided into short paragraphs with key words capitalized, often paired with a visual, such as a photo of whales during a marine biology lesson, to bring the topic to life.

As the coach reads, they may spell out complex words to help Sam process them. To an outsider, Sam might seem distracted—looking away or repeating lines from a favorite video. Still, when he spells "DOING HARD PUZZLES TAKES MENTAL GYMNASTICS" after a lesson about an unsolved mystery, it's clear just how much he's taken in.

Recently, Sam started reading lessons aloud himself. His words can be hard to follow without the text. But hearing his voice tackle the material, shifting from what looks like passive disengagement to full expression, I'm overcome with gratitude and admiration.

After reading, Sam answers a carefully sequenced set of questions designed to build his confidence, from simple recall to full self-expression.

—

The Structure: From Known to Open

The questions follow a careful progression to build Sam's confidence, guiding him from simple recall to original thought, with each step becoming a small victory.

Here's how it works for Sam:

- **Spell Words:** Sam spells capitalized keywords from the story. For example, "OCEAN" from a marine biology lesson helps focus his motor planning and attention.
- **Knowns:** A direct question with one clear answer from the story—"What country was mentioned?" — "BRAZIL."

- **Prior Knowledge:** A question from Sam's existing knowledge. For example: "What state do you live in?" — "CALIFORNIA."
- **Semi-Opens:** A question with multiple correct answers from the story—"Name one animal seen at the zoo." — "ELEPHANT."
- **Prior Knowledge Semi-Open:** A question drawing on general knowledge—"Name a U.S. state by the ocean." — "FLORIDA."
- **Emerging Open:** A question from Sam's own mind—"What's one word you think of when you hear the word snail?" — "SLIME."
- **Full Open:** The goal is to produce a completely original thought—"What is something you want to achieve?" — "REALLY WANT TO LEARN NEW SKILLS SERVING OTHERS."

This thoughtful system is more than a spelling lesson. It's a scaffold for liberation. Each stage builds Sam's autonomy, expression, and connection—another step toward sharing a voice that's always been there.

Real Words *with* Sam

The bitterness of cacao seeds is an excellent evolutionary adaptation. What is an adaptation you have?

I'M LISTENING EVEN WHILE TALKING

Name a concern you think regular folk wrestle with?

LIFE IS NOT EASY
STRESS TAKES TOLLS ON PEOPLE
MONEY TOUCHES EVERYONE

In one sentence explain why you think the author stated that poor is eternal.

THE REAL RICHNESS ISNT
RELATED TO MONEY
YOU MIGHT BE RICH BUT POOR IN SPIRIT

Why do you think rich dad said they would learn faster in the real world?

REAL WORLD TEACHES MORE TIMES TEN

What are your thoughts on what makes someone a monster?

THE UTMOST DISRESPECT
FOR OTHER PEOPLE AND HARMFUL ACTION

What makes a good role model?

ONE TRAIT IS INDEPENDENT THOUGHT

Chapter 6
Nice to Meet You, Sam

It happened in a rare moment of quiet, almost casually. But my fundamental understanding of Sam shifted.

Not suddenly. Not dramatically. In fact, it felt somewhat routine.

Sam was working through his usual steps—spelling key words, answering known questions—when his coach added one more.

A different kind of question.

The kind we'd talked about just days earlier.

And without hesitation, Sam spelled his answer.

For about a year, he'd been meeting with his spelling coach once a week. The rhythm was familiar. The sessions steady.

But that moment was different. And it moved something deep inside me.

When Sam first started, it was hard to imagine we'd get here.

Some sessions were rocky. Dysregulation, distraction, frustration.

There were times I wasn't sure if spelling would ever really click.

But as he grew more comfortable with his coach, and with the process itself, something started to take hold.

His body began to cooperate. Intentions finally turning into action.

And at first, I was just amazed he could spell the words from the reading paragraphs. That alone felt like a breakthrough.

His coach would say something like, "Spell *environment.*" And Sam would slowly, carefully point to each letter:

E - N - V - I - R - O - N - M - E - N - T.

I don't think I ever took that for granted. Watching him do that was incredible. He wasn't just parroting; he was attending, tracking, decoding, spelling. Every letter was intentional.

But then, several sessions in, he started answering questions.

Not just spelling pre-selected words, but responding with a single, meaningful word.

I remember one day his coach asked, "Who were the four Beatles?"

J - O - H - N   P - A - U - L   G - E - O - R - G - E   R - I - N - G - O

I don't think I've ever been more proud.

After that, we listened constantly to the Beatles station on Sirius XM. He loved it—I know because he'd tune to it himself.

If you ask him, "Who's the greatest rock band of all time?" he can give you an answer—and it's the right one. To be fair, he is also a huge fan of the Beach Boys and Jimmy Buffett.

For months, he stayed in that phase—keywords and one-word answers. It was steady, slow, and honest work. In every session, the pattern was the same: Read, spell-words, known questions, semi-opens…

But then we reached something new.

There's a type of question in the spelling community known as an emerging open.

It's not yes or no.

It's not multiple choice.

It's not drawn from the text.

It's the kind of question that asks the student to reach inside themselves and say something only they could say.

That's where spelling moves from skill . . . to voice. Not just letters anymore. But language that belongs to him.

The day it happened for Sam, the topic was something about activities people enjoy.

I don't remember the exact story.

But I'll never forget what came after.

His coach asked, "Sam, what's something you like
to do?"

We waited.

Letter by letter, slowly and with purpose, Sam spelled:

"RELAXING IN AN EASY CHAIR"

We laughed.

We cried.

We sat there stunned.

Not because it was poetic or dramatic.

Because it was real.

Because it was his.

We've never used that phrase around our house.

We say recliner. Maybe La-Z-Boy.

But "easy chair"? That came from him—maybe
something he picked up from a movie or TV show, or a
book read years ago.

But that's the thing.

He picked it.

He stored it.

He reached for it.

And he used it—not just to answer a question, but to
show us that there were whole worlds inside of him we had
never accessed before.

It wasn't the sentence itself that shook us. It was the
fact of it.

We'd spent more than a year spelling. Hours of regulation, focus, effort, and repetition. And then, we heard our son express a fully original thought for the very first time.

And in that moment, something clicked open inside of me.

Any trace of cautious belief disappeared.

This wasn't just a method. This was Sam.

Not a behavior. Not a collection of challenges. Not a mystery we'd never solve.

A thinker.

A person.

A son I was only beginning to truly meet.

Real Words *with* Sam

Name an instrument.

THE DRUMS

Name one more.

THE TROMBONE

What does the Bible say about creation?

ALL THE STUFF IN THE WORLD
WAS MADE IN ONE WEEK

What is the effect of smoke on bees?

IT SUBDUES THEM

What's your smoker that subdues you and makes you feel calm and in a happy place?

HELPING OTHERS DO LIFE

What's the honey in your life that sustains you and drives you forward?

RELY ON THE UNDERSTANDING THAT YOU
BELONG TO THE LORD

Chapter 7
Looking Through Glass

It's not that he wasn't welcome—though it sometimes felt that way.

Our church lacked the resources and trained staff Sam needed.

And truthfully, very few churches in our area did.

So when we found North Coast Church in Vista, a place with a class designed for children and young adults with special needs, we exhaled.

For the first couple of months, he mostly stayed off to the side.

He didn't participate.

When it was time to stand for singing, he stayed seated.

When the teacher began a story, he acted disinterested, doing his own thing.

He still spoke constantly, repeating words and phrases that looped through his mind.

But he caused no disruptions.

He was present—part of the room, but not quite part of the moment.

Until one Sunday, he decided to do something different.

It wasn't gradual.

It wasn't a series of small steps.

One week, Sam was still sitting in the corner.

The next week, he took over the class like he'd been leading it for years.

He set up chairs.

He cued the video at the exact right moment.

He stood at the front and helped lead the singing.

Nothing happened without his steady hand.

He had absorbed every rhythm, every cue, every expectation—and when he decided it was time, he stepped straight into the center of it all.

Years later, when he'd become a fixture in that classroom, one of the teachers told me how much they'd missed him the Sunday he was gone.

"I couldn't even remember how to run the video," she said, laughing.

"Sam usually just handles it."

That's him.

HELPING OTHERS DO LIFE

In a thousand ways.

One particular Sunday, as I stood behind the glass and watched him move through his routine, something stirred in me more than usual.

I stepped away, pulled out my phone, and wrote this reflection—part poem, part prayer:

Wet Eyes and Lessons

(By Sam's Dad)

I watched him open the door and enter the class.

He greets his teachers with enthusiasm and joy.

Some kids are playing with toys

I can see through the two-way glass.

Tears begin to form in my eyes as I watch my boy.

It's not sadness;

But a feeling hard to explain.

Maybe they're tears of gladness,

Because it seems that he feels no pain.

I don't think he knows he's so different

Than most children his age.

Truth is, he's heaven-sent.

In God's unfolding story,

Sam's life is my favorite page.

His innocence shines brightly

As he gives his teacher a cheek kiss.

She hugs him back tightly.
My heart kinda flutters.
My wet eyes, impossible to miss.
One of my favorite things to do each week
Is watch him on Sundays through that window.
What I see and the reports I hear later
Are of an angel on Earth.
Without judgment, he loves all.
We can learn something from Sam
Perhaps no lesson greater.
He teaches us by his actions.
I pray we answer that call.
Sam inspires me to love life and love people
At all times. In all places.
Not just under a steeple.
Since so many families don't get to have
A blessing like our little mister,
Maybe this poem can help
Somehow, some way.
So from me, his dad,
And his beautiful mom and awesome sister:
Embrace life with unconditional love
And have a happy, hugs- and- kisses day.

Years later, I still find myself watching through glass.

Not the glass of a Sunday School window anymore—but the kind that forms from my own assumptions.

I used to assume he wasn't paying attention.

That he was lost in his own world.

That if he wasn't responding, he wasn't connecting.

But that glass has been shattering piece by piece.

I see now how much he absorbs. How much he contributes.

How much he leads, with flair, focus, and zero apologies.

And again and again, I'm humbled by what I see.

Real Words *with* Sam

What genre of literature peaks your interest?

STARTING TO DEVELOP AN
INTEREST IN ART

What does it mean to admire something?

TO SEE ALL THE BEAUTIFUL PARTS

What other adjective would you use to describe Venice?

ARTISTIC

What is your opinion about what it would be like to live in a city that requires water transportation?

THE ADVENTURE TRAVELS
WOULD BE A SWIFT REAL RIDE

Give your own synonym for "victory".

WIN

Why do you think they chose the name Nike after the Greek goddess of victory?

STRONG NAME TO PREDICT
A VICTORIOUS FUTURE

Chapter 8
The Long Way Home

Today was hard.

And meaningful.

Sam's full-time aide was out sick, and so was the backup.

So I took him to school and stayed for the day.

My to-do list was waiting. None of it mattered more than this.

We left on time and even arrived a few minutes early. A good start.

First on the agenda today: motor skills class—basically PE.

We stretched, did some yoga and body-weight exercises, then hopped on treadmills side by side.

We did a mile, followed by a short meditation.

It was a little loud, but Sam and the others handled it well.

After that, we had a break.

He ate a snack. We took a breather—just relaxed, no rush.

Then came group spelling, and things began to unravel.

The room was noisy.

The lesson: Earth Day.

Sam nailed the spelling words, but then hit a wall.

Six simple questions, one-word answers straight from the lesson—a chance to get into a flow.

He stared, tried, fidgeted.

Not one answer down before the class moved on. A new paragraph, a new round of questions.

Too fast. Too noisy. Too much.

He didn't handle it well.

Louder. More frustrated. Less regulated.

By the end, he was shouting, distracting the others.

After class, everyone left the room, but we stayed.

We reread the paragraph with fewer distractions and got through four or five questions. But he was still anxious, talking loudly about computers at home, the fire drill coming on Friday, and how he didn't want his lunch.

After forty-five minutes of minor progress, another class arrived, and we gave up on the assignment.

He marched to the restroom, tossed his lunch in the trash, poured out his drink, and we left. We needed air. Distance. Movement.

Reading this now, it sounds easier than it was—but in real time, it stretched my composure thin.

To wait him out.

To be present.

My patience wore down. My blood pressure rose more than once.

If I—who know and love him deeply—felt my patience slipping, how much harder must it be for someone who doesn't know him like I do?

After school, we drove around.

At first, just to cool off. And it worked.

But then it became something more.

We stayed out for more than two hours, driving along the coast, through new neighborhoods, taking the scenic route.

Christian music played softly—peaceful, grounding.

No real destination, just movement. Just time.

He rubbed my shoulder and spoke softly. "Be nice to Dad," he whispered.

By the time we got home, he was grounded again.

As challenging as it was, I'm filled with gratitude.

Today didn't go as planned, but it brought us closer.

I was where I needed to be.

And I wouldn't trade that for anything.

Some days undo us.

Then make space for something better.

Real Words *with* Sam

What is a physical task you would be willing to endure to achieve a goal that is important to you?

PRACTICING TYPING WITH BOTH MY DAD AND MOM TO BE ABLE TO SAY LOADS OF THINGS IN EVERYDAY MOMENTS

What qualities or attributes are most important to you in a 1:1 coach?

A DESIRE TO GET TO KNOW THE REAL ME AND A BALANCE OF UNDERSTANDING AND PATIENCE

What do you want your 1:1 Coach to know most about you or your wants/needs/hopes?

TO KNOW THAT SAMUEL LONGS FOR A COMMUNITY ABOUT TRUE INCLUSION WHERE I CAN THRIVE BEING MYSELF AMONGST LIKE MINDED INDIVIDUALS

Is there anything that you would like to add?

THAT I LIKE TO RUN WITH MY OWN IDEAS BUT I THRIVE WITH A GENTLE PATIENT ENCOURAGEMENT

There are several members of a ship's crew. Name a role you think you would be good at?

THE CAPTAIN SUITS ME BECAUSE IT REQUIRES LEADING WITH DIRECTION

Chapter 9
Time To Spare

Getting out the door is part of the journey.

If we need to leave by 11:30, I start the process early. Sometimes the day before, sometimes even earlier.

Sam needs time to prepare, not just physically, but mentally, too.

I might tell him, "Sam, we need to leave at 10:00."

I know we don't really need to leave until later.

But if I say 10:00, we might, through a familiar mix of patience and persistence, land somewhere closer to 10:30. If he agrees to 10:30, we'll probably leave closer to 11:30.

The negotiation is almost a ritual.

If I say, "We need to leave at 10:00," Sam might immediately counter: "Two o'clock."

I'll explain why that's too late.

"One o'clock," he'll try again.

"No."

"12:00."

Back and forth we go, our usual give-and-take.

Eventually, with enough patience, we'll agree on a time, often 30 minutes after the original proposal. He needs to feel like he won the negotiation.

But even then, the time we agreed on isn't when we actually leave.

It's just when he starts getting ready.

Getting ready means three things:

Brushing his hair.

Brushing his teeth.

Putting on his shoes.

When the agreed time comes (say, 10:30), if I'm not paying attention and a few minutes slip by, he'll notice.

If it's 10:33 and he's in the middle of a video, he'll say, "Finish the watch," asking for a few more minutes.

Whatever the new time is, rounded up to the next five or ten, becomes the new goal.

So 10:30 might stretch to 10:35. Then 10:40. Maybe even 10:45—always a multiple of five.

If he can, he'll try for 11:00.

Our best chance of leaving close to on time is when I give him countdowns, like stepping stones to departure:

"Two minutes, Sam."

"One minute."

"Time to go!"

Even then, it's not guaranteed.

But it helps.

And if I build that time in, if I plan for it, we can leave without stress, and do what we set out to do.

Sam and I both love public transportation.

When we go bowling, we walk to the bus stop, catch a bus to the transit center, then take the Coaster train for a quick ride to Pacific Coast Highway.

From there, it's a short walk to the bowling alley.

Sam carries his own bowling ball and shoes, tucked inside a bag with a strap slung over his shoulder.

And, he insists on carrying my shoes too, in a separate bag.

(That's Sam HELPING OTHERS DO LIFE— another one of my favorite revelations he shared with us.)

When we arrive, we set a time to pick a lane.

If we get there at 1:15, we'll agree on a time, "At 2:00, we pick a lane."

At 2:00, choosing a lane begins—and that can take a while.

It's not that Sam doesn't know which lane he wants. I think he knows the moment we walk in. But standing at the counter, getting his body and words to align with what his brain has already decided? That part can take time.

It might be thirty minutes past our agreed-upon time. Other days, longer. Once, it was over two hours.

It's not always easy to be patient, but I've learned not to rush the process. We'll get there.

So I wait.

Sometimes reading a book.

Sometimes scrolling through messages on an iPad.

Sometimes just watching the world move around us.

You might wonder why we let him pick.

Usually, when you go bowling, they just assign you a lane.

But years ago, a friendly desk clerk gave us the choice, and that set a precedent.

Now, Sam has to pick his own lane.

If I try to pick for him, or let them assign it, there's a battle, and it's usually loud.

So we work together, patiently, until he's ready.

And he picks odd-numbered lanes.

Except once.

In more than fifteen years of bowling together, he picked an even-numbered lane a single time.

I still don't know why—Maybe something to do with three cute girls in the next lane.

Then again, I don't really know why he prefers odd-numbered lanes at all. Maybe it's keeping the ball return on his right, easier for his dominant hand to grab.

Sam's actions may seem random, but there's almost always a reason.

A wise parent or caregiver, through observation, patience, and experience, might figure it out about 25% of the time (if the clues line up just right).

We usually bowl two games each. Yesterday, I won the first game; Sam claimed the second. (He wins more often than I do.) The scoreboard doesn't lie, but it also doesn't capture the real victories—the patience, the waiting, the small celebrations between frames.

Packing up is easy.

Maybe because he loves public transportation. But that doesn't seem to help him leave the house promptly. Another mystery.

We pack up our bags, wash our hands, catch the train back to the transit center, ride the bus to the stop near our house, and walk the last mile home.

Another day together.

Another odd number chosen.

Another small, shared victory.

One five-minute increment at a time.

Real Words *with* Sam

Why did the kings agree to stop war?

THEY BELIEVED THAT THE OLYMPIC
GAMES WERE MORE IMPORTANT THAN
THEIR RIVALRY

What do you imagine the audience was like at an ancient
Olympics?

ABSOLUTE CHAOS A FRENZY OF EXCITEMENT

Give me one word you think of when you think of surfing?

BADASS

What do you think it takes to become the most
accomplished surfer of all time?

ATTENTION TO THE LITTLE DETAILS SUCH
AS BEING AWARE OF THE WAVES AND BEING
ABLE TO READ THE CHANGING OCEAN

THEN IT REQUIRES PERSISTENT PRACTICE
AND THE INNER DESIRE TO KEEP
PROGRESSING

What does it mean to be in your prime?

ARISING TO LIFES PEAK TO LEARN THE BEST
MOMENTS ARE HAPPENING RIGHT NOW

What qualities would make an athlete have a long career
in their sport?

PASSION AND FRIENDS WHO
SUPPORT THEIR DREAMS

Chapter 10
Full System Reset

The spelling session had completely fallen apart.

His mind was engaged—you could see it in his eyes. But no rhythm took hold. Not with the lesson. Not with the spelling. Not with the cadence he depends on.

He didn't get far that day.

His coach tried everything: spell words, gentle encouragement, simple questions. Nothing stuck. In spelling, when the body won't sync with the mind, nothing moves forward.

Eventually, the clock ran out. Sam put away his letterboard and marched out the door, overwhelmed and visibly frustrated.

But then something happened.

As he reached the car door, his agitation peaked. He paced back and forth a few times, repeating two words—louder, more insistent each time:

"There's more . . . there's more . . . there's more."

Intense and purposeful, he broke away from the car and headed back to the building

He wasn't missing anything.

He was resetting.

There are times he has to return—physically, mentally, emotionally—to where he started.

When he does this, it's as if his mind insists on a clean slate. A full-system reboot. Not distraction or avoidance. But orientation and order. A deliberate return to the beginning so he can move forward with purpose.

By returning to the car, back to where the session began, Sam was starting over.

Once back inside, he picked up the letterboard, placed it in his coach's hand, and began to spell.

Not in response to a prompt.

Not because someone asked.

But because he had something to say.

TIME REALLY NOT MY ALLY

I NEED MORE TIME TO BE REGULATED

TEN TONS OF PRESSURE WEIGHS ME DOWN
WHEN THERE ARE LIMITS TELLING US WHEN
TO START AND STOP

MY PLAN IS TO LEAP INTO GROWTH
THROUGH SPELLING

This wasn't just about a hard session.

It opened a window into how he experiences time, pressure, and hope.

And for the rest of us?

It was a lesson.

Sam was showing us something deeper—something true for all of us.

In life, we often find ourselves off track.

We're overwhelmed.

Behind.

Lost.

When that happens, our first instinct is to course-correct quickly—to push through the discomfort and keep going.

Now and then, that works.

But not always.

At times, the only way forward is to stop—to back-track, to return to the place where things first slipped off course, and begin again, with new intention.

Sam does this instinctively.

And in doing so, he reminds us:

Starting over isn't failure.

It's clarity.

It's courage.

It's strength.

In Sam's words, it makes space for a LEAP INTO GROWTH.

Real Words *with* Sam

Unprompted:

CAN TIME STOP ORDERING ME AROUND

If you were to live in a similar harsh environment, what would you do to survive?

WEAR A SUIT OF ARMOR TO WITHSTAND THE TEMPERATURES AND THE PREDATORS

If you could have armor, what would it be like?

MY ARMOR IS MADE OF SPARKLE GOLD MORE FLASHY THAN FUNCTIONAL

How would you define introspection?

TRYING TO INSPECT UNCONSCIOUS PATTERNS GOING ON INSIDE YOURSELF

What do you want to achieve?

REALLY WANT TO LEARN NEW SKILLS SERVING OTHERS

MIGHT I ADD THAT CORE TIME SPENT WITH MY FRIENDS IS ALSO IMPORTANT

Chapter 11
The Gardener

Silence.

We didn't get much of it when Sam was awake.

But after he fell asleep, when the house was dark with only the hum of the ceiling fan, we sat with silence often.

Not in confrontation. Not in despair. Just silence.

The kind that settles in when two people are trying to figure out something for which they are unprepared. Staring at a patch of soil, minus a green thumb, hoping something will grow.

Developmental delays.

Therapies.

Treatments.

Timelines.

Early interventions. Seeds scattered in uncertain soil; costly, exhausting, and none of it guaranteed to help.

No fighting.

No harsh words.

But the silence between us often felt heavy, like something we didn't yet know how to carry.

There's a quiet truth that shadows families like ours:

Raising a child with autism can put enormous strain on a marriage.

Some studies suggest divorce rates 50% to 100% higher than average.

The risk is higher.

The toll is heavier.

And the weight doesn't lighten with time.

There's pressure.

Grief.

Financial stress.

Therapies. Travel. Testing.

Much of it out-of-pocket.

And no way of knowing what may make a difference.

No wonder so many marriages don't make it.

Marriage is hard under the best of circumstances.

Add autism: the cost, the uncertainty, the constant adapting. It gets harder to stay connected.

Harder to stay present.

Harder to stay you.

But for us, the strain never fractured.

Paulette and I have been married for thirty-one years.

And every now and then, someone asks us what the secret is.

What keeps us going, still grounded, still together.

We never know quite what to say.

We've never had a screaming match.

Never gone to bed mid-argument.

Never raised our voices at each other—not once.

That's not some kind of marital heroism.

It's wiring.

She's intense in all the best ways.

I'm even-keeled, maybe too even sometimes.

And by the grace of God, through decades of faith and commitment, we've walked in rhythm, even when life felt anything but rhythmic.

Still, that doesn't mean we carried the same weight.

Especially in the early years.

When it came to Sam's development, therapies, challenges, and his path forward—

Paulette carried more.

A lot more.

She did the hard stuff and some of the easy stuff.

I did some of the easy stuff and none of the hard.

While I stood on the edge of the field, she had her hands in the dirt.

But I never stood in her way.

If she said, "I want to try this therapy," I didn't question the price or the method.

If she said, "Let's fly across the country to see a specialist," I didn't push back with logic or doubt.

I knew this wasn't my wheelhouse.

I didn't understand the therapies, the diagnoses, the alphabet soup of acronyms.

I'm wired to solve problems with logic and reason. For a long time, I didn't think those tools applied to Sam.

So I stepped back.

Not out of disinterest, but because I trusted Paulette's instincts more than my own.

I showed up in the ways I knew how.

But I didn't give her enough hugs.

Didn't ask enough questions.

Didn't sit beside her in the dark as often as I should have.

That's not some overblown confession—it's just the truth.

She was holding up the sky, and I was mostly watching.

I wasn't physically gone.

But emotionally? I often was.

Not cold or cruel. Just distant, avoiding the soil.

And if you asked Paulette whether I was loving and supportive during those years,

I'm not sure she'd say yes.

Because I wasn't leading.

Not in the strategy.

Not in the advocacy.

Not in the day-to-day effort of guiding Sam forward.

I told myself I was working.

And sometimes I was.

But more often, I was retreating: into a screen, into a project, into the quiet safety of my home office. Building just enough justification to let someone else carry the heavier part of the story.

That someone was Paulette.

She read the books.

Attended the conferences.

Took the late-night notes.

Wrote the emails.

Tracked the research.

Talked with other parents.

Drove the long miles to doctors who might, somehow, hold an answer.

She planted.

Watered.

Pruned.

Observed.

Adjusted.

Waited.

A gardener who stayed with the soil even when it looked dry, trusting the seedling long before it showed signs of life.

And that's one of the hardest parts about raising a child like Sam:

You can do everything right—all the interventions, all the research, all the therapies—and still not see the blooms you hoped for.

We watched other kids, once so similar to Sam, develop language.

Gain independence.

Leap forward, while our son's progress stayed largely hidden.

Sam showed little progress on the surface.

His growth came in tiny ripples, not waves.

Hidden. Subtle. Sometimes invisible.

And when nothing seemed to grow, it would've been easy to walk away from the garden.

To say, "We've done all we can."

To stop expecting fruit from barren soil.

Paulette didn't.

She kept tending.

Kept believing.

Kept kneeling in the dirt, trusting that the roots were doing something no one could see.

She treated Sam as whole.

Never lowered the bar.

Never made excuses.

Never made him feel like one, either.

She believes in good manners. So if he forgot his in public, she didn't wave it off.

She'd offer a quick, calm redirect and say, without flinching,

"He can be autistic, but he can't be rude."

That blend of compassion and accountability has been one of the greatest gifts she ever gave him.

That unwavering belief—that Sam was in there, learning, absorbing, becoming—was the truth she never let go.

And she was right.

Sam's mind—brilliant, observant, articulate—was growing all along.

Apraxia masked it, but it was never absent.

His body couldn't keep up with his thoughts, but the thoughts were there.

Always there.

They were preserved—nurtured—because she stayed in the garden even when nothing seemed to grow.

I helped now and then.

Maybe I held the hose or handed her a trowel. Small things, while she did the real tending.

Tilled the soil.

Monitored the shade.

Watched the weather.

And she never walked away from the garden.

—

A Truth That's Hard to Say

I've taken Sam on weekend getaways. The easy stuff, at least compared to what Paulette was doing.

I stayed home with Sam while she traveled across the country for conferences, trainings, and therapies we hoped might unlock something new.

We've gone to the beach. To amusement parks. On short cruises.

I've had moments of being the fun dad. And those moments matter.

But if we're measuring time, energy, emotional labor, especially in Sam's younger years, it wasn't close to even.

Maybe 90/10.

Maybe 95/5.

And while I never disappeared, I wasn't the one charting the course.

I wasn't the one making the map.

Paulette was.

She didn't check out.

She didn't stop hoping.

She didn't let go of the idea that Sam's story was still unfolding.

And because of that, she stayed in the fight.

And because she did, Sam grew.

Not suddenly. Not obviously. Not like many others.

But steadily. Gently. Deeply.

He grew into the young man who now spells profound truths.

Who thinks and can write like a poet.

Who reflects with nuance and grace.

That didn't happen randomly.

It happened because someone believed in the seed—long before anyone saw the bloom.

—

Setting Up the Stories Ahead

There are dozens of stories I could tell about Paulette's strength.

Moments where she held the line when everything felt like it was slipping.

Moments when her intuition beat out all the experts.

Moments when love looked like research, or a spreadsheet, or a confrontation, or a 3 a.m. prayer.

In the next three chapters, I'll share just a handful.

They're not polished.

They're not easy.

But they matter.

They shaped Sam's life.

And they helped shape the family we've become.

And one day—maybe—she'll write her own version of these stories.

But this is what I saw.

This is what I know.

But first, of course, some more Real Words with Sam, then a few stories from the garden.

Real Words *with* Sam

What inspires you?

MY FAVORITE INSPIRATION IS MY PARENTS

Name one thing you would want to be sure to have with you on your tour of the Washington monuments?

MY PARENTS AND A MAP OF THE
MONUMENTS TO KEEP US ON A TOUR
OF THE MUST SEE SIGHTS

What is one thing that is a treasure?

A TREASURE IS THE SUPER STRONG
CONNECTION THAT I HAVE WITH MY MOM

What is a quality you look for in a leader?

I LOOK FOR MOM LIKE LOYALTY

In your own words, summarize what bravery in the midst of chaos means?

TO PRESS ON DESPITE EXCESS TURBULENCE
THAT MIGHT CAUSE FEAR OR UNCERTAINTY

Chapter 12
Footsteps to Freedom

Of all the mountains Paulette has climbed, this one was the steepest.

"It was the hardest thing I've ever done in my life."

That's what she says even now—decades later.

Not childbirth. Not the maze of doctors and diagnoses. Not surviving years of sleep deprivation.

This was a mountain where every step was hard-earned.

Potty training.

Sam was four years old. Still in diapers.

Paulette had done the research, spending late nights scrolling through message boards, medical sites, obscure forums—any place where desperate parents like her were searching for hope.

Any method. Any story. Any sign that a kid like Sam could learn this.

After months of searching, she found something that felt different—a specialized program developed by a university in Southern California. It wasn't even designed for kids. It was created for adults with significant developmental disabilities who were in adult diapers.

That's how specific it was.

And how serious.

The program didn't come with a binder of protocols or a step-by-step playbook. It came with a thin, stapled pamphlet, just a few folded pages with a narrative overview, a basic checklist, and minimal instructions. Paulette had to extrapolate, improvise, and figure out how to make it all work at home.

One detail still stands out—not from the program, but from Paulette's own playbook. She had Sam stand on a sheet of paper so she could trace his feet.

Then she copied the outlines, cut them out, and taped them to the floor—left foot, right foot, left foot, right foot—from every room in the house to the toilet.

My job? I took Madison to Texas to visit family. We were gone for 10 days. I left like a backup singer skipping out while the headliner continues on stage alone.

While Madison and I were eating BBQ and Tex-Mex, trying to stay distracted, I was still getting updates from Paulette.

Text at noon: *'Small progress.'*

Text at midnight: *'I can't do this.'*

I knew she was drowning, but from Texas, I couldn't truly grasp how deeply she was buried.

Meanwhile, Paulette stayed home, turning our house into base camp. She became a full-time, round-the-clock potty training sherpa, hauling all the weight while guiding Sam toward a summit she believed he could reach.

I can only imagine what those 10 days were like. Every moment had to be structured.

Every ounce of energy focused.

It was a battle of attention, timing, resistance, and pure grit.

The program required absolute consistency. No breaks. No wavering. Just reset after reset, day after day—each one another uphill step on the same unforgiving mountain.

The house was filled with defiance, determination, and a whole lot of laundry. A cycle of accidents, resistance, and bodily fluids—parenting's greatest hits.

There were surely moments when giving up would have made sense.

But Paulette had already made the decision: there was no exit ramp. No plan B.

Just this path, and her determination to see it through.

We'd cleared the calendar. Cleared the house. This was happening, no matter how steep the climb.

And she did it.

She made real progress during those 10 days. However, it still took the entire summer for everything to fully take hold. This included educating Sam's preschool teacher on the process and staying in the classroom for a few days to ensure the follow-through was successful.[2] And Sam learned. The impact wasn't immediate, but it was permanent.

Many parents can relate to the idea of investing time upfront to teach a child something that will pay off for years to come, such as learning to tie their own shoes. It takes effort. It takes patience. But once they've got it, you're no longer tying their shoes every morning.

This was like that, but a thousand times harder.

Dialed to 11.

Set to a soundtrack of screaming.

All the pressure and none of the gratitude.

Most of what Paulette did was invisible. There was no applause. No breaks. No backup. Just her—gripping the rope and climbing anyway, even when the summit felt impossible to reach. Her investment, her discipline, her patience, her refusal to give up gave Sam something that now feels ordinary: independence in the restroom. No supervision. No anxiety. No need for help. That may sound like a small win to some.

For families like ours, it's monumental.

---

2   Paulette had to teach the school teachers and support staff to say "restroom" rather than "bathroom." For literal thinkers like Sam, matching the word to what's actually written on the door removes one unnecessary confusion.

That single skill has preserved his dignity, enabled him to travel, and allowed him to attend school, church, restaurants, and theme parks. It has made life so much easier for all of us—but, more importantly, for him.

And the credit goes to the one who stayed behind.

Feet planted, path marked.

Walking him, footprint by footprint, toward a freedom most people take for granted.

Real Words *with* Sam

What is a feeling someone might have at the end of the training?

SATISFIED

Name part of the brain?

THE PARIETAL LOBE

Imagine that you could create a planet out of anything, describe what your planet is made of, and what it is like?

MY PLANET IS MADE OF COTTON CANDY
THE GROUND IS SOFT

If you could communicate with any animal which would it be and why?

I WOULD COMMUNICATE WITH WHALES
BECAUSE THEY COULD CARRY MESSAGES
ACROSS THE OCEANS

In your own words, what does it mean for something to be cryptic?

CRYPTIC MEANS TO BE CONFUSING

What is something about yourself you think people admire?

NURTURING SIDE
VERY NICE TO FRIENDS

Chapter 13
Bon Appétit

He screamed as the fork flew across the room.

Behind the two-way mirror, Paulette stood frozen, heart pounding, feeling helpless. In the next room, a determined therapist was doing her best to help Sam eat a single bite of squash.

She wasn't succeeding.

This wasn't a tantrum. This was a war.

And food was the battlefield.

At 18 months old—when the regression hit, when his speech began to disappear, when the stomach issues started, Sam self-selected down to five foods and refused everything else. His world of food shrank: pretzels, Goldfish, bacon, rice, and grapes. That was it. He used to eat more.

For more than a year, we watched Sam live on that tiny menu. Paulette knew that couldn't last. Not just for nutritional reasons, but because she could see it: Sam was trapped. Limited by a body that resisted what it needed most.

So she did what she always did: she researched. She found a clinic in Tarzana that specialized in cases like Sam's—kids whose bodies resisted food in ways that weren't about choices but wiring.

We didn't know the name for it at the time.

To us, it felt like stubbornness.

Most people would think the kid is spoiled, defiant, or just being a pain.

But it wasn't that. It was apraxia affecting his eating, just like it affected his speech and movement.

And while we understand that now, we still don't always know when to push, when to pause, or how to stop blaming ourselves or him, for battles we don't fully understand.

This wasn't a fix for picky eaters. It was for kids with full-blown sensory aversions—some who'd nearly stopped eating altogether. The method was intense: controversial, confrontational—and just maybe, life-changing.

She packed for a week: clothes, nerves, and the essentials she always carries. Faith, hope, and love.

Then she took Sam to Pasadena to stay with our friends J.P. and Anne, commuting each day to the clinic.

Five days. Eighteen sessions. All focused on eating.

Madison and I stayed home. Paulette carried the hard part—she always did when Sam needed something we didn't yet know how to give.

Paulette emailed friends and family: *"We've tried to get him to eat in the past, and it didn't go so well. The likelihood of gagging, vomiting, screaming, food throwing, and who knows what else is likely. I'm holding out for some surprising blessings. Sam may surprise us, and God might, too."*

Even as I describe it now, I wrestle with how it felt. Necessary on one hand, but deeply unsettling on the other. The clinic's method was simple and brutal: pick a toy, lose the toy, earn it back by taking a bite. And if Sam didn't choose? They would physically introduce the food. Yes, force feeding: holding his mouth open and placing food inside. Paulette compared it to something some parents can relate to:

"This is like putting your kid in drug rehab. It sucks and it's painful, but it's the right thing for the possibilities of the outcome."

There were bright moments. In the early sessions, Sam picked out toys, paired them with foods, and even swallowed a green bean. But there were also hard, heartbreaking hours.

"I was on the third floor in the elevator, Sam was on the second floor, behind closed doors. I could hear the screaming. He is not cooperating at all. I hear forks flying and yelling for me. I stayed out of the room for the first half hour." After going back and watching through a two-way mirror, she added, *"I should have stayed out!"*

Later: *"He is a kid you just have to wear down constantly so that he knows he's not getting his way. 'No!' is the word of the day…"*

The next day: *"I felt your prayers yesterday. I was ready to pack it up and head home. Sam tried to pack us up last night and drag everything to the van; he cried himself to sleep, bless his heart. This morning, same thing. But once we got here, he was excited because he got to play in the elevators! Up and down yesterday for maybe an hour and a half straight. Cheap entertainment."*

It's hard to describe how I felt during this process. On one hand, I could feel the weight of Sam's suffering: his confusion, his exhaustion, his tears. But in many ways, Paulette's burden hit me even harder. She was the one in the trenches, facing the screams, the mess, the decisions, the mirror of her own doubts.

While I don't really believe in guilt the way most people describe it, something in me still wrestled with that. Could I have done more? Maybe. Maybe not. Maybe this was the way it needed to be. What I do know is this: I had complete faith in Paulette's resolve, her discernment, her love. If there was anyone I trusted to walk Sam through the fire, it was her.

What haunts me now is that I didn't know that Sam was completely aware, processing all of this fully. What did he think as food was being forced into his mouth? Was he resentful? Sad? Angry? Confused? Or did he somehow understand, even then, that he needed to eat more than five things, that his long-term health hung in the balance? We were making decisions about his body while assuming his mind couldn't grasp what was happening. Now I know better. He understood every moment, but did he grasp why?

With more spelling proficiency, I expect we will be able to "talk" about it. I'm curious about so many things…

That week, Sam added new foods: peas, waffles, apples, carrots, and even a few bites of squash (after a fight).

From five foods to more than twenty in that first week. From refusal to tolerance. From chaos to choice. Paulette carefully kept track of what worked and what didn't.

"I know we have a long way to go until it looks normal. I'm not even sure what 'normal' looks like. I'm hoping he's capable of getting there so we can eat as a family without it being so clinical."

Paulette often wondered if meals would always feel like a fight, or if one day, eating could just be eating. Not strategy. Not structure. Just food and family. No more short-order cooking. Just one meal we all share.

The program didn't end when they got home; it just changed locations.

In another email, Paulette wrote:

"Poor Sam . . . When we're doing the eating program, he says, 'Go home.' Even though he is home. I think his saying 'Go home' is like saying, 'Hey, what happened? I thought that was over. I have to eat this stuff at home now? Well, this just bites!'"

"Go home," he yelled, again and again, even though they already were. It wasn't about location. It was about escape.

Thinking back on this now, maybe 'Go home' really meant 'Go back'—to before food became a battlefield, before eating meant fighting his own body.

Paulette held the line and willed it forward.

Today, Sam mostly eats what we eat, though he still resists new foods. We've found our rhythm. I'll set something on the side of his plate. Most of the time, he ignores it. Sometimes he moves it. Every once in a while, he tries it.

And when he does? That's a win.

A win made possible by a mom who believed her son could grow—and believed it hard enough to endure the screaming, the flying forks and food, the sessions, the structure.

And the squash.

That freedom wasn't given.

It was fought for, one bite at a time.

Bon appétit.

Real Words *with* Sam

The Beach Boys and a Breakthrough

In one of his college classes, Sam gave a presentation on his favorite music. He opened by playing a short video clip from a tailored spelling session created specifically for this class project:

Do you want to do your assignment on The Beach Boys?
SAFE TO SAY THAT IS A YES

What do you like about The Beach Boys?
ALL THEIR MUSIC TRANSPORTS ME TO A RELAXED AND EASY LIVING MINDSET

Anything else you want to share about The Beach Boys?
THE ISLAND ROCK UNWINDS MY TENSE MIND AND USUALLY HELPS ME TO FEEL THE EASE OF THE BEACH BOYS LIFESTYLE

Then, to complete the assignment like everyone else, Sam sang karaoke.

His song of choice? "Help Me, Rhonda."

He crushed it!

It was a breakthrough moment. Most of Sam's classmates are highly verbal. He rarely speaks in class and has never been able to show them the depth of his mind.

But in fifteen minutes, that changed.

The energy in the room transformed.

His classmates, professors, and aides were wide-eyed, many in tears, and gave Sam a huge ovation—and their respect grew tenfold.

Sam held his head higher that day. And has been picking up good vibrations ever since.

Chapter 14
Big Hugs

My wife is a hugger. Not a quick-pat, half-squeeze kind of hugger. She hugs with her whole heart—and you feel it, whether you're ready or not.

Now, full disclosure: I've become more of a hugger over the years. Not naturally, but inevitably. When you live with someone like her long enough, hugging starts to feel less like a gesture and more like a duty of the heart. Some say I give decent hugs now, even if most are still one-arm, sideways efforts. But the obvious credit goes to Paulette. She turned me.

So when our son Sam started pulling away from touch, it hit hard. He didn't just resist hugs. He shrank from them. He cringed when we got too close. His nervous system seemed to short-circuit at contact. For a mother whose love poured through her arms, it wasn't just heartbreaking. It felt like exile.

But Paulette, the gardener, didn't accept that.

She'd kneel beside him and say, gently but firmly, "I don't know what's going on with your brain right now, but I'm going to hug the love into you." Or sometimes, "You may not like it, but I'm going to love you through it anyway."

She found her way in. Slowly. Stubbornly. One careful cuddle at a time.

Resolve. Not strategy.

A mother choosing to show up with love, even if he turned away, flailed, fussed, or melted down halfway. Even if it looked like rejection.

Sometimes it was a hand on his back. Other times, a full-body hug mid-protest. Or a kiss on the head with both arms wrapped around him while he squirmed.

She didn't wait for permission. She gave connection anyway. He's all boy, after all, and roughhousing is its own kind of affection.

Over time, she brought touch back, reframing it not as something he owed her, but as something she owed him. A constant. A truth that didn't change based on mood or meltdown: You are loved, even when it's hard.

Watching it unfold, I didn't know if it would work. I didn't overanalyze. I just watched and respected. I saw her persistence. I saw the way she showed up, again and again, even when it didn't seem to make a difference.

Over time, it did.

Even now, Sam hugs his mom and his granny more than he hugs me. Some envy creeps in, I'll admit.

I usually just ask for a lean (head to chest, no arms).
The dad version, I guess. I'll happily receive what's offered
and honor the path it took to get there.

These days, Sam hugs freely—sometimes too freely.
The barbershop incident is one example of hundreds. We've
learned to say 'Three . . . two . . . one...' to help him release.

But watching him embrace the world with open arms,
I see what Paulette planted: more tolerance for touch and
a connection that took root, sprouted trust, and slowly
bloomed into a heart that knows how to love back.

Real Words *with* Sam

What is one way that you like to celebrate?

SINGING HAPPY BIRTHDAY

Name one word that comes to mind when you think of a cactus?

SHARP

How would you describe the feeling of descending into complete darkness, going to the bottom of the ocean?

LIKE YOU ARE BEING LOWERED INTO THE OPENING OF A GROUP OF SEA MONSTERS PREDETERMINED TO EAT YOU

What would you do if you discovered evidence of a lost civilization?

SPREAD THE MIRACULOUS NEWS AND TAKE ALL THE CREDIT FOR MY DISCOVERY

Name something that brings bad luck according to some?

A SILLY MYTH STATES THAT BLACK CAT SIGHTINGS ARE BAD LUCK

What inspires your thirst for knowledge, and why?

CULTIVATING A TROVE OF INFORMATION KEEPING ME FRESH AND HOT ON WHAT IS HAPPENING IN THE WORLD IS A GO

Chapter 15
Birthday

I get to be here with my son. That matters more than the fact that today, Sam turns 24.

We're sitting outside his school—just the two of us, a small table, a little patch of grass, and some trees.

He's watching the cars go by, smiling.

I'm watching him, learning more about who he is, what lights him up, how he thinks, how he connects.

It took us a while to get to this moment today.

Little comes quickly or easily, but it comes.

And when it does, it's worth the wait.

Some days are loud and full of repetition.

Some are long and full of resistance.

And we are both here for each one.

Even when it's hard, I wouldn't trade this time with him for anything.

He's teaching me patience, presence, and joy in the simple things.

That's the real celebration.

Happy 24th, Sam.

I'm honored to be your dad.

Real Words *with* Sam

What is one object that may be polished in a house?

SILVERWARE

If you were a toy designer at this time, and all you had was wood, clay, and bone, what toy would you design?

LIFELIKE TAIL TO USE AS A COSTUME

Name a sound you might hear on the bridge?

THE SOUND OF ROAD TRAFFIC
TONS OF CARS HURRYING ACROSS

What would you set out as an offering for your deceased relatives?

ON THE CHRISTIAN RITUAL OF FUNERALS
WORLDWIDE RULERS LEAVE FLOWERS

Would you like to write a message to your dad for Father's Day?

TO SPELL OUT A MESSAGE FOR MY DAD
WOULD SURELY BE THE BEST

Message for your dad for Father's Day?

DEAR DAD WITH FATHER'S PROTECTION
NOTHING CAN HARM ME

THANKS DAD, PARENT EXTRAORDINAIRE
YOUR SON, SAMUEL

Chapter 16
Superpower

Before I knew the word "stim," I saw it in action.

The hand flapping.

The rhythmic rocking.

The repeated sounds.

The fixations on specific movements or words.

For Sam, it's often triggered by motion—credits scrolling on a screen, cars passing outside a hotel room window, trains, planes, and roller coasters.

He really likes roller coasters.

He can watch them for hours, sometimes on YouTube, sometimes in person. Not even riding them—just watching: the climb, the drop, the loops, the blur of motion.

He loves the patterns, the predictability, the flow.

And sometimes, as he watches, his body echoes the excitement—flapping, rising up on his toes, stiffening his shoulders back, wringing his hands, voicing a long, drawn-out vowel—stretched and repeated, over and over again.

They're called stims, short for self-stimulatory behavior.

They're common in many people with autism, especially children, and they're not random.

They serve a purpose, often more than one.

As Dr. Barry Prizant writes in *Uniquely Human*:

"Many autistic people engage in repetitive behaviors, called 'stimming.' These behaviors serve an important purpose. They can help regulate anxiety, express excitement, or simply bring comfort. It's not meaningless. In fact, it's often the opposite—a coping mechanism for navigating a world that feels overwhelming."

Stimming isn't always something that needs to be fixed.

But it can be exhausting.

For Sam, it's not always something he wants to be doing.

Sometimes it's something his body does, even when his mind wants something else.

During one of his spelling sessions, his coach asked him a creative, open-ended question:

"If you could choose one supernatural power, what would it be?"

Sam answered:

SUPERPOWER IS TO STOP STIMS BECAUSE THE TIRED STIMS NEED TO LET UP

That sentence . . . wow.

There's so much in it.

The awareness. The exhaustion. The wish.

It tells me that stimming isn't always joy.

Sometimes it's pressure. Sometimes it's compulsion.

Sometimes it's simply too much.

And it reminds me: just because something looks repetitive doesn't mean it's easy.

Or even wanted.

Sam's answer isn't dramatic.

It doesn't come with tears or raised voices.

But in that one sentence, he gives us a window into the tension he lives with every day—between what his body demands and what his heart desires.

His answer wasn't about flying or invisibility.

It was about stopping suffering: his own, and others like him.

When given the chance to wish for anything…

he asked for peace.

It makes me rethink what a superpower really is.

If that's how Sam sees it (not flashy or grand, but necessary and kind), then maybe the rest of us already have a few superpowers of our own.

Small ways to ease someone's struggle.

Quiet moments where we choose compassion.

Choices that don't make headlines, but change someone's world.

Maybe that's the kind of power that matters most.

Real Words *with* Sam

What is something Mrs. Claus might learn at the school?

HOW MUCH TRAINING IT TAKES TO LEARN
THE ROAD TO BE MARRIED TO SANTA CLAUS

In your own words, what is a cryptozoologist?

A PROFESSIONAL RESEARCHER OF
THE FANTASY

Use the word elusive in a sentence.

THE HUNT AFTER THIS ELUSIVE
BEAST REMAINS

HOW TIME BODES ON THE EAGER
OUTSIDE HUNT

Use sophisticated in a sentence.

HARDLY SOPHISTICATED IN REALITY
IM SUCH AMERICAN

Do you consider yourself more of an idealist or a realist
and why?

I AM MORE OF AN IDEALIST BECAUSE LIFE
INSIDE MY HEAD IS PLAYFUL

If you could choose one supernatural power, what would
it be?

SUPERPOWER IS TO STOP STIMS BECAUSE THE
TIRED STIMS NEED TO LET UP

Chapter 17
The Distance Between Us

Not everything that looks random . . . is.

Among the many myths that linger around autism, this one is among the most damaging:

The idea that certain behaviors—their movements, actions, choices—are meaningless.

It's not true.

Not for Sam.

Not for so many others.

Sure, there are times when an action is purely sensory: when Sam wrings his hands with excitement, or echoes a phrase from VeggieTales, Wonder Pets, or even Wheel of Fortune, just for the pleasure of the sound. That's part of who he is.

But it's not always just repetition for comfort.

Sometimes, Sam uses those familiar words to communicate.

It reminds me of Bumblebee from the Transformers movies, the robot whose damaged voice box forces him to communicate through radio clips.

Bumblebee can't speak directly, so he uses snippets of radio broadcasts to express what he's feeling or needing.

That's what Sam does sometimes, too.

He can't always summon brand-new words easily.

So he reaches into the library of words he already has, pulling out a phrase that fits (or almost fits) what he's trying to say.

Sometimes, if I listen closely, I can hear the difference—a little more emphasis in his voice, a phrase repeated more insistently, a deeper urgency beneath the surface.

The challenge for me is recognizing when he's just enjoying the rhythm of language . . . and when he's really trying to reach me.

I can only imagine how frustrating it must be for him to work so hard to send a real message, only to be misunderstood or missed altogether.

But I've learned (usually the hard way) that when something doesn't make sense to me, it's not because Sam is random.

It's because I'm missing the message.

Sam is constantly communicating, just like the rest of us. And here's the thing:

Because of apraxia, every successful message Sam sends out is a victory of perseverance on his part. There's a reason behind every gesture, sound, or sequence of movements.

Sam is working hard to reach me.

To reach anyone willing to listen.

Maybe not always with words, but with his actions, body, and choices.

The question isn't whether he's trying. He's trying with everything he's got.

The question is whether I'm listening.

Over time, I've learned to approach these moments like a puzzle:

Not with frustration, but with curiosity.

Not demanding that Sam explain himself, but asking: *What is he trying to tell me? What does he need that I'm not seeing yet?*

It's not his job to bend himself into a shape that's easy for me to understand.

It's my job to slow down, pay attention, and listen with all the tools I have.

Communication is a two-way street.

And when I remember how hard Sam is working to send his message, I realize:

The least I can do is walk my half of the distance.

Real Words *with* Sam

What iconic landmark would you be interested in visiting?

ALL OF THEM

What word describes how you might feel walking into the
White House?

ABSOLUTELY READY TO CONQUER
THE OVAL OFFICE

What is an item you would hope to discover on an
archeological dig?

ANCIENT BOOKS UNDISCOVERED BY MAN

Summarize what fueled Jeffrey's passion for Eagles Autism
Foundation.

BROTHER LOVE IS A POWER I DARE
NOT ATTEMPT

Give one to two words that you would use to describe your
brain?

ABSOLUTE CREATE NEW TERM FOR MY
KIND OF BRAIN

What does it mean to hypothesize?

IT MEANS PREDICTIONS IN
NORMAL SCIENCES

Chapter 18
The Phantom At Tea Store

And just like that, he was gone. One second, he was walking the sidewalk like we'd done dozens of times before. The next, he turned a corner, and vanished from sight.

This wasn't new. Since Sam could walk, he's been a master at disappearing, earning the nickname *The Phantom*. One moment he's beside us, the next, he's gone. Paulette and I learned fast: in public, we can't chat for long without a glance, our hearts always half-braced for his next vanishing act.

A steady sweep of glances, always watching, like radar tracking a fleeting blip that is Sam, slipping away to chase his own quiet plans.

He wasn't reckless. He didn't bolt into traffic, though his unpredictability meant we always had to stay alert. But he could slip silently into a nearby aisle or storefront like it was a magic trick—gone before we even realized he'd moved.

Now that Sam's in his 20s, I try to give him more independence. He's an adult. But without a reliable way to communicate with the world, his feet and his behavior often had to speak for him. At the time of this story, spelling wasn't yet a part of his toolkit. His "voice" was his movement, his patterns, his persistence.

We don't let him roam the streets completely alone. Paulette's heart still skips anytime he's out in town without me right beside him, her quiet worry echoing his phantom ways.

So, Sam and I found a rhythm. Two or three times a week, after hitting the gym, he'd walk to a nearby spot. Maybe a burger joint or store, while I trailed in the car, leapfrogging parking lots like checkpoints, my eyes on him, my heart balancing trust and caution.

It gave him independence. It gave me a sense of control. Until it didn't.

At first, those walks were just a block or so, close enough for me to shadow him on foot. But as his confidence grew, so did his range. Two blocks became a half-mile, then became more. That's when I started driving from lot to lot, playing a quiet game of automotive tag.

Sometimes he'd get in the car and ride home after our stop. Other times, he'd want to keep walking the rest of the way home, another couple miles. I didn't want to risk a three-mile round-trip on foot just to retrieve the car. So, leapfrog it was.

That day before the gym, in his determined voice, Sam kept saying, "The at tea store." Our verbal exchanges were like decoding invisible ink, waiting for the right light to reveal its truth, one I'd soon uncover.

I figured "the at tea store" was Sam's code for the Albertsons grocery store we often visited. Just a new shorthand for a usual stop. I didn't think twice.

But when Sam locks onto an idea, he doesn't let go easily. He'll ask sixty, seventy times a day—sometimes more. That's not hyperbole. Parents of children with autism know exactly what I'm talking about. It's persistence, yes, but more so a pattern. Involuntary. A loop his body gets stuck in, even when his brain might want out.

And yet, it's also a kind of fire. The kind of energy that pushes through resistance. That doesn't quit. If most people had even a fraction of that force, they'd blow past their goals in half the time.

So we went to the gym. We worked out. Then we walked outside, and the routine resumed. He hit the sidewalk, and I got in the car to tail him.

I parked, watched him pass, then eased ahead. Stopped again. Waited. Watched. Our familiar dance of independence training.

Until I didn't see him.

Traffic in the parking lot held me in place longer than anticipated. By the time I moved, Sam had rounded a corner, gone. I knew his pace, his paths. He wouldn't stray.

I turned the corner, expecting to see his familiar stride in seconds.

He wasn't there. My chest tightened.

Okay. No panic. I ran through the mental checklist: he's probably headed to the grocery store. Makes sense. I drove to the store, parked, and stepped inside in search of the phantom's trail.

I checked both grocery entrances, asked around—nothing. My heart quickened. I widened the search, hurrying to the pharmacy, its automatic doors a magnet for Sam's delight. No dice.

Ten minutes had passed. Then twelve. My heart had moved from casual stroll to light jog, each beat slightly more urgent than the last.

I darted into every storefront in the strip mall, my steps quickening. Then I stepped into the cell phone store. My heart exhaled in relief. There he was.

Sitting calmly, exactly where he wanted to be, completely absorbed in an iPad display. The employee behind the counter looked up, smiling. "Is he with you?"

I exhaled a laugh. "Yeah. He's with me."

"He's been here about five minutes," she said. "He's doing great."

We were lucky that day. The clerk smiled. Sam was calm. Everything went fine. But it could've gone another way.

When they are young, the world is more forgiving. But when they grow up and look like adults who "should know better," the world can become less patient. More punishing. And when communication breaks down, misunderstanding can be dangerous.

We've all seen the headlines. The wrong move, the wrong assumption, someone calls the police. A young man like Sam, moving unpredictably or repeating words too loudly, might seem threatening to someone who doesn't understand.

But what looks like defiance is often just a body trying to stay regulated—or a brain stuck in a loop it didn't choose.

I nodded, took another look at Sam, and then the lightbulb moment landed. He'd been telling me all day. The at tea store wasn't some grocery shortcut.

It was the AT&T Store. Sam knew exactly where he was headed all along. I thought I held the reins. But he is the one with the plan, even when the rest of us don't under-stand him.

That moment stuck with me. Long before spelling unlocked his brilliant thoughts, before I understood that "at tea" was actually *A-T-&-T*, Sam was already showing us something else: he knows what he wants. He knows where he's going. He just needs the tools and ears to be heard.

It repeated the lesson of how often we misread hearts—not for what they lack, but for what we assume. I'm learning to see beyond my own blind spots.

Sam wasn't lost. I was. And every day beside him, he leads me around corners I didn't know existed.

Real Words *with* Sam

How do you think the world would change if everyone experienced a communication disorder?

I THINK PEOPLE WOULD BE MORE
KIND AND UNDERSTANDING

If you could, how would you change the world?

I WOULD CHANGE HOW ALL PEOPLE
VIEW THOSE OF US THAT CAN'T RELY ON
OUR BODIES

TIME AND EDUCATION SHOULD HELP PEOPLE
SEE THE TRUTH

What is something important you want people to see in you?

AN EDUCATED WORLD VIEW
LIKE MY PARENTS

Imagine you are an author of children's books. What phrase might you use to end your books?

STEAL MOMENTS OF JOY

The text talked about how Loki has a dual nature. Share what that means to you.

THE LIKE OF LOKI SHOWS US THAT
PEOPLE HAVE MORE INSIDE THAN JUST
ON THE SURFACE

What does success look like to you?

THE TERM SUCCESS MEANS HAVE MORE EASE

The next four chapters follow a day in Sam's life.

We'll start at the end with *Bedtime Prayer* and work our way to the beginning.

Chapter 19
Bedtime Prayer

There was a time when prayer was something we did for him. Now it's something we do with him. Or maybe more accurately . . . something he lets us share.

No matter what kind of day it's been, Sam ends it the same way—calm, still, and reverent.

There's a stillness in him that's hard to describe unless you've seen it firsthand. Quiet surrender.

When we reach this moment, something has shifted. It's like peace moves in, and it's always welcome.

He begins the same way every time:

"Dear God . . . thank you…"

And then comes the list.

"Uncle Austin. Uncle Bruce. Uncle Mark. Uncle Steve."

"Aunt Suzanne. Aunt Barbara. Aunt Christie. Aunt Sandy. Granny and Pal." "Michael Lemaster. Mr. Tyson."

"Madison and Grant"

It started with a few names. A couple of uncles and aunts who were facing health concerns or specific challenges. We'd ask Sam if he could pray for them, and he did. Night after night. And then, as loved ones entered seasons of need, we added a name here, a name there. Eventually, the list settled into what it is now.

Some beloved family members didn't make the list—not because we love them any less, but because in Sam's world, once the rhythm is set, it rarely changes. We've tried adding a few more in recent years, but it seems like Sam has reached his limit. So for now, the list is closed. But the ritual continues.

After the last name, there's a little sound he makes, tough to explain but unmistakable if you've heard it. The closest thing I can compare it to is a burst of static on a walkie-talkie after someone finishes talking. Sam's way of saying, *"over."* Like the prayer has been sent, and now he's waiting for God's reply.

After the transmission is sent, he launches into *The Lord's Prayer.* We say it out loud together, honoring his mother's Catholic background.

"Our Father, who art in heaven, hallowed be thy name…"

He's always reverent. Sometimes he speeds through it—like his mouth is hurrying to keep up with his spirit. But we keep pace with him. Whether it's just me, or Paulette, or all of us, this part we say in unison.

I don't just listen. I participate and remember how far we've come.

He walks around the foot of the bed. Turns off the light. Slides under the covers, pulling them all the way up over his head—all while speaking:

"It's bedtime."

"Lay down on my pillow."

"We're tired."

"Good night, Dad."

"See you on Sunday."

Or Monday. Or Thursday. Whatever day comes next.

Not always in that order. Not always just once. But always some version of it.

Then comes my part. I sit beside him and pray out loud. I thank God for the day, for our family, for health and rest. Sometimes I mention something that came up that day—something that felt hard or beautiful or worth carrying into sleep. I talk with God about gratitude, blessings, grace, and opportunity. I know Sam and God both listen.

When I finish, I gently pull the covers down from over his head. That's his signal. He lifts his chin, just slightly, inviting the kiss on his head I'm about to give.

"Good night. You are my favorite Sam. I'm so proud to be your dad. I love you."

Sometimes he lets out a soft, warm sigh—like he's exhaling the last tension of the day. I pat his side and stand up.

I echo one of his earlier phrases, *"See you on Sunday,"* and quietly step out. The door clicks closed. The hallway light goes off. And somehow, all is well.

Even on the hardest days, this blessing endures.

Real Words *with* Sam

Name something that is priceless and cannot be bought
with money.

IT IS CERTAINLY PRICELESS THE TIME WE
GET TO SPEND AWAKE

How might you feel if you saw a ghost?

PROBABLY SCARED BUT EXHILARATED

Would you ever live a state that has experienced a
hurricane and why?

REALLY PREFER TO STAY SAFE ON
THE WEST COAST

What would you do if you came face to face with a dinosaur?

SCREAM AND RUN

Would you like to see dinosaurs roaming in the present
day? Why or why not?

ONLY IMPOSSIBLE TO HAVE THEM ROAMING
AMONG US WITH NO DANGER

What quality do you admire most in explorers or scientists?

INTELLIGENCE MOTIVATION AND DRIVE TO
CONTINUE LEARNING MORE

What is one gift you offer the world?

OBSERVING TINY DETAILS AND HOLDING
THEM IN MEMORY IS ONE OF MY STRENGTHS

Chapter 20
The Evening Routine

Before prayer time, there's a routine that helps Sam settle in. It's not dramatic or complicated, but it's consistent. And that sameness seems to be what makes it work.

It starts with shutting things down—screens, the ceiling fan, maybe a couple of windows if they've been open. Sometimes Sam kicks it off without a word. Other times, he needs a little prompting. I never know if he'll ease into it on his own or try to squeeze out a few more minutes before winding down.

He walks to the kitchen and opens the dishwasher. Loads the soap. Closes the door. Pushes the button. We don't ask him to do it—it's just part of his rhythm now. I have to believe that powering down the house helps him power down his body.

He gets a big plastic cup, fills it with ice, and carries it to the bathroom, setting it beside the shower.

He gets undressed at his own pace. The last thing to come off, every time, is his watch.

While all this is happening, he's talking. Loudly.

"It's shower tiiiime!"

"Look, Dad—the dishwasher is on!"

"Take my clothes off!"

Once he steps in, the first thing he does is wash his face. He has used the same soap since his early teens.

He calls it his *"washing my face."* A prime example of a message we had to decode.

When it runs out, he lets us know.

"More washing my face, Dad."

There's pride in it, not in the soap, but in the act of doing it.

There was a time when we had to wash his face for him, scrub his body, and wash his hair. But, over the years, he learned to manage the routine mostly on his own. He's capable. And he knows it.

After that, he moves to the ice. He takes a few pieces from the cup and holds them under the hot stream. One by one, they melt in his hands.

Cold fades.

Solid softens.

Eventually, there's nothing left but warmth.

I've never asked him why. I don't think I need to.

Something about it calms him. Maybe it's sensory or just the routine.

Whatever it is, he emerges more steady, inside and out.

But the ritual isn't complete.

Then comes the pause.

After washing and melting the ice, he just stands there, silent under the water.

Not moving. Not in a hurry. Just letting the moment stretch—sometimes for half an hour or longer, unless we gently prompt him forward.

And what's he doing?

Watching the water run down the glass.

Replaying something from earlier.

Imagining what tomorrow might bring.

Maybe he's simply letting his mind go quiet for a while.

And I want to let him enjoy those minutes.

Most nights, someone will have to say something to spark the next phase.

"Go ahead and wash your hair."

And usually, within thirty seconds, his head goes under the stream.

That's the trigger.

Once the hair is wet, the rest is automatic.

The shampoo is rinsed, and with that, this part of the evening routine is complete.

No more prompting. No more delays.

He's on his own rails.

By the time he steps out, the shift is nearly complete.

Body relaxed. Mind settled.

Whatever was happening in there, it worked.
Because once he gets to bed, sleep comes easy.
We meet in his room for prayer.
One rhythm ends. Another begins.
And with it, the day lets go.

Real Words *with* Sam

What is an innovator?

SOMEONE WHO TALKS INTO HIS PATENT
RESULTING IN SOMETHING NEW

What is one emotion that boxing fans might feel while watching a fight?

AROUND SO MANY OTHER ENTHUSIASTS THE
PEOPLE LIKELY FEEL COMMUNION

If you had to choose between the fields of science, education, and politics, which would you pursue and why?

EDUCATION BECAUSE THE WORLD
NEEDS TO UNDERSTAND HOW TO TEACH
NEURODIVERGENT MINDS

What would you consider the secret ingredient to a long and happy life?

TO LEARN THE LESSON THAT EACH PERSON
IS CREATED TO LIVE A UNIQUE NEVER
DUPLICATED LIFE AND TO ACT ACCORDINGLY

Summarize the Japanese concept of "ikigai" in your own words.

EXPLORING YOUR IKIGAI MEANS TO
PINPOINT WHAT MAKES YOU LIGHT UP

THIS LOOKS DIFFERENT FOR EVERYONE

Chapter 21
What Time Is It?

For two decades, I thought I understood Sam's love affair with time.

I was wrong.

Time isn't just Sam's oldest obsession—it's his most complicated relationship. And like so much about my son, I'm learning to see through his words before I see through his eyes.

Every morning, Sam straps on a watch with the precision of a pilot checking instruments before takeoff.

He loves watches. Wears one every day. Picks it out with care.

He narrates the clock like a sports announcer. He knows what day it is, what's coming next, and how many days until the next holiday.

And yet, he once spelled something that made me rethink all of it.

Something that suggested time might not feel like a friend after all.

How do I make sense of that?

We feel fortunate that Sam can dress himself—and he does it with a bit of flair. His ability to coordinate colors is impressive, especially considering he's also matching his watch.

Sam doesn't just wear watches—he curates them. Thirty-six so far, stored in five sleek watch boxes like artifacts in a museum. Most cost under twenty-five bucks, but that misses the point entirely. Each one chosen, worn, and remembered—evidence of a mind that treasures order and beauty.

He's proud of his collection.

Picking the right watch isn't random. It's part of his morning ritual.

He chooses with intention. The color has to match his shirt. And when we travel, he packs a different watch for every day we'll be gone—carefully matched in advance.

Each morning, Sam announces (several times, never quietly):

"I got my clothes on!"

"My watch is on my wrist!"

Sam doesn't just check the time.

He narrates it.

It's not just about what time it is. It's about what time it's almost.

"It's almost 9 o'clock!"

That declaration starts at 8:31—the countdown begins.

Then, at 9:01, the next one starts: the march toward 9:30.

He lives in that in-between space, anticipating the next marker, sensing the shape of the day through the numbers on his wrist. We don't lose track of time when Sam is home. Between any two markers, he might call it out fifteen times.

He tracks the calendar this way, too.

Always forward-facing. Always counting down.

"Today is Thursday, June 26. Five more days 'til July."

Then he might rattle off, *"July, August, September, October, November, December! Six more months!"*

We learn about holidays from him, too.

"Today is Boxing Day," he'll declare. Or Passover. Or Watermelon Day.

He doesn't need a planner. He practically is one.

And he's got a fun party trick.

When we're hanging out with friends, I'll ask someone, "What's your birthday?"

They'll say, "November 15."

I turn to Sam, and he knows what I want—the day of the week.

At first, he'll often default to *"No."*

But then, he closes his eyes…

Pauses for a few seconds…

And delivers the answer: *"Saturday."*

He's rarely wrong.

Even if it's next year.

It feels like a magic trick. But of course, it's not.

Maybe he's memorized the calendar for the year ahead. Is he calculating in real time?

The method matters less than what it reveals: Time has been his thing since he was a young boy. His ally. His anchor.

Which is why his words, when they finally came, stopped me cold:

CAN TIME STOP ORDERING ME AROUND

…and…

TIME REALLY NOT MY ALLY

TEN TONS OF PRESSURE WEIGHS ME DOWN
WHEN THERE ARE LIMITS TELLING US WHEN
TO START AND STOP

What do I do with that?

For years, I believed I understood Sam's relationship with time—the comfort it brought him, the predictable rhythms, the reliable structure. But then he spells those words, and suddenly I'm seeing it through his eyes.

The very thing that anchors him
also chains him.

I look forward to the day when we've practiced enough spelling to have full conversations, so I can ask him about these things directly.

Until then, the best I can do is let him select his watch each morning—this ritual that both grounds him and burdens him.

Every day, he chooses his anchor. Every night, he sets himself free.

Such a small act. But like most things with Sam, it carries the weight of mysteries I'm still learning to understand.

Real Words *with* Sam

I, Sam Britton, am passionate about ____

SO MANY THINGS

Like?

WATCHES

If you could ban something what would it be?

LYING TO YOUR PARENTS

If you were prince for a day, what would you do?

ENTER SCHOOL RIDING A HORSE

What does inclusion mean to you?

INCLUSION MEANS TO NOT LEAVE
US TRUSTING AUTISTICS OUT OF
INSTRUMENTAL SITUATIONS

Unprompted:

CAN TIME STOP ORDERING ME AROUND

TIME REALLY NOT MY ALLY

I NEED MORE TIME TO BE REGULATED

TEN TONS OF PRESSURE WEIGHS ME DOWN
WHEN THERE ARE LIMITS TELLING US WHEN
TO START AND STOP

Chapter 22
A Day in His Rhythm

The negotiation started the night before, as it always does.

"What time to get up?" He'll ask.

He doesn't really want me to answer. He wants me to ask it back. If I offer a time, I'll get an almost automatic, *"No."* But if I mirror the question, he'll begin the dance.

"Six o'clock, Dad."

Sam doesn't sleep in. Even if he's up late, he wants to get up by 6 a.m.

If I counter 8 a.m., he won't split the difference and settle at 7.

He might concede ten minutes at first.

Most nights, we land around 6:15 or 6:30.

It's not a battle worth fighting.

—

There's no such thing as a normal day. Not really. Not for anyone.

There are patterns and rhythms we fall into. But normal? That's a word for someone who isn't paying attention.

Still, the idea is worth exploring. So I'll do my best to capture it.

When it's time, he's up. No alarm needed.

He emerges fully dressed. Socks on, no shoes.

To the first person he sees:

"Look, Mom, the clothes is on."

He doesn't say it once. He says it a dozen times in the first hour. Not a question or request. It's a declaration. A signal that the day has begun.

And with that signal, Sam begins his rounds.

On days without a scheduled program or outing, Sam settles into a familiar rhythm.

The house fills with layered soundtracks from screens in three rooms.

In the Sam Cave, he keeps multiple devices running—laptop, portable DVD player, and an old VHS player he's maintained through sheer force of will. I hunt down VeggieTales and other tapes on eBay like an analog archaeologist.

The VeggieTales aren't just background noise. Sam catches the wordplay, the biblical parallels, the jokes within jokes. He gets the layers.

In the master bedroom, Sam finds something familiar: Wheel of Fortune, Arthur, Super Why. He sits for 30 seconds of theme song, opening credits, and he's gone, only to reappear for closing credits. He either has a timer in his head or an uncanny ability to hear things happening across the house. Probably both.

Meanwhile, in the kitchen, a smartphone plays a rollercoaster ride or an airplane window view—some stranger's iPhone video uploaded to YouTube, now part of Sam's daily rhythm.

He patrols between screens like he's checking on old friends. Rarely sits long. But each screen, each sound, holds a piece of comfort. A thread of control.

I've learned that control matters to Sam. And nowhere is this more obvious than in his ownership of household tasks.

He does all the laundry. Every load. Every day. Even if there are only two dirty items, he wants to wash them. We've had to regulate load sizes to conserve water and electricity, but his commitment doesn't waver. He loads, washes, dries, and hangs everything. Fridays are for towels. Other days are assigned by person. Madison brings her laundry over weekly, and Sam handles it with pride.

He also takes out the trash and recycling. If someone else beats him to it, he's not thrilled.

Same goes for the mail. The walk to the mailbox isn't far, maybe thirty yards, but it matters. If someone else gets it first, he'll protest. He delivers the mail back to the box, waits a few minutes, and retrieves it himself. Because to him, this job needs to be his.

There's meaning in the motion. More than being a helper, he's claiming responsibility. Participating in the life of the household. On his terms.

Throughout the day, between chores and screens, Sam takes time to connect with whoever's home. He'll talk about the past, but more often, he talks about what's coming next.

He'll ask about the next day.

"What do on Tuesday?"

Me: "School on Tuesday."

"Wednesday."

"School."

"Thursday." "Friday." "Saturday."

If I say something that's not set in stone.

"Saturday, let's go to Legoland."

He'll shut it down.

"No, Dad. Washing my clothes."

I should've learned by now. He's not really asking because he wants an answer. He'd rather I repeat the question back and let him say what's on his mind. He craves predictability.

Control.

And generally speaking, he doesn't want to be asked questions. Not the way most people do it. It feels like an interrogation.

"How was school?"

"Do you like that pizza?"

"Do you remember me?"

Maybe he answers one or two. But by number three, it's almost always curt:

"No."

And he leaves the room while well-meaning people smile like they understand.

But Sam's need for connection runs deeper than answering yes or no questions, doing chores, and following routines. Between the screen rotations and household tasks, he seeks us out.

That's when new questions enter the mix—ours, not his.

Should we try a spelling lesson today? Maybe some schoolwork?

Should we disrupt the rhythm of the screens? Get him out of the house?

Tension creeps in.

We know Sam wants to spell. He's told us, in his own words, that he's willing to work hard for it.

When asked: "What is a physical task you would be willing to endure to achieve a goal that is important to you?"

He spelled:

PRACTICING TYPING WITH BOTH MY DAD
AND MOM TO BE ABLE TO SAY LOADS OF
THINGS IN EVERYDAY MOMENTS

But that's not the same as agreeing to a lesson at 1 p.m.

If we say, "Let's do 30 minutes of spelling," we'll likely hear one of three responses:

"No spelling today."

"Sorry, Dad. Maybe next time."

Or, jaw clenched, shoulders tight, and five notches louder than necessary:

"Zero minutes!"

Sometimes it takes hours of nudging just to begin. And by the time we get there, he's so wound up that it's hard to get much out of the session.

And sometimes, after all that pushing, we don't get there at all. Which leaves us with a hard question:

Is it worth it?

Is the push worth the spiral? The shouting? The tension it brought into both of us?

And yet, when we don't push, when we let him drift between screens, what communication have we missed? What growth have we passed by? How many beautiful conversations could've been unlocked if we'd just pressed a little harder . . . or a little more skillfully?

It's not that Sam lacks desire. Inertia is powerful. Sam at rest stays at rest. And once in motion, he stays in motion. I've learned what works: planning the lesson at least two days in advance, and mentioning it several times so that his mind and body can prepare. And timing—first thing in the morning, before the screens begin their pull. Once the electronics start, the window closes. But at 6:30 a.m., when the house is quiet and his mind hasn't yet scattered across three rooms . . . that's where possibility lives.

If we can gently help him shift toward engagement, inertia starts working in our favor. On his best days, once the lesson begins, he locks in. He might spend 90 minutes or more reading, answering questions, and working through homeschool assignments. He's finishing two classes for his high school diploma: Bible and personal finance. Those days are rare. And I have to admit, I've probably contributed to that inconsistency.

Here's a hard truth I live with: the path of least resistance for Sam is also the path of least resistance for me. Letting him do what's easy is easier for both of us. And my early reluctance to press through that resistance has made it even harder now.

Like most dads, I have a long list: people to call, chapters to write, and things that feel urgent. Do I really have time to carve out three hours for something that might not produce any visible result—something that almost certainly brings anxiety, frustration, even borderline anger to both of us?

In those moments, I return to Dr. John Trainer's words: "Children are not a distraction from more important work. They are the most important work."

I carry those words each time Sam approaches me with anything he has to say. (Here's irony: several times while writing this chapter.)

I know it's not easy for him to initiate conversation.

Still, it takes concentrated effort and discipline to stop what I'm doing, turn, face him fully, and be nowhere else.

"…the most important work."

—

By evening, whether we've pushed through resistance or given in to it, Sam settles back into his most predictable rhythms.

At 6:00 p.m., he turns on the news. Not because he's interested, but because years ago, Granny told him she likes to watch it at that time.

After the news, it's Wheel of Fortune. Then maybe Jeopardy, but more often it's The Big Bang Theory.

He doesn't always watch. But he knows the rest of us enjoy the clever writing and quirky characters. Maybe that's why he keeps them playing—his way of contributing to the mood.

As the evening settles around us, Sam begins his own settling ritual.

Sometime between ten and eleven, he starts shutting things down. Electronics off. Dishwasher loaded and humming. The transition has begun.

From there, we move into the evening ritual and bedtime prayer.

I don't have it all figured out. Not even close.

But I'm paying attention and leading with presence.

The day ends.
Reflections.
Challenges.
Blessings.
Gratitude.
"What time to get up?"
The cycle continues.
Hard day? Normally.
Normal day? Hardly.

Real Words *with* Sam

How can the staff best support you with your schedule rigidity?

DO RUN THE SHOW EVERY DAY THE COACHES DO NEED TO COACH ME MORE FIRM

What does being proactive mean to you?

TO TAKE ACTION WITHOUT NEEDING TO CATCH INSTRUCTIONS

If you had to choose between either of those professions, which would you choose and why?

I THINK I COULD BE A GOOD CRYPTOGRAPHER BECAUSE MY MIND SEES PATTERNS

What is one strength you have that could help in a chaotic situation?

STARTING MOVEMENT WITH PURPOSE

Are you interested in using the letterboard or typing in future sessions?

ALL THE FUTURE SPELLING VISIONS I MAKE FOR MYSELF INCLUDE TYPING

Who is known as the Lamb of God according to John?

JESUS

Chapter 23
Different Classrooms

I was sitting in the back of a conference room, listening to Jeff Bry read from his journal about his son's summer job. I expected to smile and nod. Instead, I found myself fighting tears.

He spoke with pride about his son's growth—the confidence gained, the grit developed, the lessons learned through a summer of selling. Jeff shared about the first day his son, Logan, made phone calls, moving from scared and grumpy to "Hey, this is kinda fun." It was heartfelt and familiar. The kind of story I'd heard hundreds of times over three decades with Vector Marketing.

But this time . . .

Jeff quoted his son, "Hey Dad, it's pretty cool being your son in the business."

A wave of emotion came fast and hard. Tears welled up. My chest tightened. And all I could think was:

Sam. Won't. Get. This.

Not because he'll choose something else. But because this choice won't exist for him.

That realization hurt in a way I didn't expect.

And that's hard for me to admit.

I'm wired to find meaning in hard things. It's almost compulsive—this need to extract purpose from pain. But every now and then, something cuts through that wiring. No lesson waiting. No meaning to extract. Just loss.

This was one of those times.

I left the room quietly. Walked the hallway for ten minutes trying to collect myself. I hope Jeff didn't take offense. It wasn't his words, but what they revealed.

I've had these moments before. At parks. At ballfields. In restaurants. Seeing kids in soccer jerseys or baseball uniforms. Watching families come in after a game, laughing over burgers. Little ambushes of what might have been.

Paulette has felt them too—even more deeply than I've allowed myself to.

This time, though, the ambush came from inside my own world. One I've been part of for more than three decades.

Vector Marketing is where I met my wife.

Where my daughter, Madison, came into her own, selling CUTCO knives right after high school, continuing through college. I watched her grow in confidence, learn to speak with poise, manage her time, and handle disappointment.

This is a world I know. One I believe in. One I've seen shape lives.

And it's not one Sam is likely to step into.

Maybe I'm lacking faith. Maybe I'm wrong. I'd be thrilled to be wrong.

But this felt like one of those rare moments where the only honest response was:

This sucks.

And I don't have a silver lining for it.

—

Later, after I'd returned to my seat, after Jeff had finished, after the day had moved on, my thoughts did not.

Vector teaches persistence. Learning not to take every outcome personally. To focus on the right activity and make small improvements every day. Showing up when it's hard.

Sam lives these lessons every day. Not in sales calls, but in trying to make his body obey his mind. In being constantly underestimated. In pushing through when his own nervous system fights against him.

He has to fight harder, endure longer to get through a single day than most of us face in a month.

He won't sell knives. But he already knows what it means to keep going when everything in you wants to quit.

Sam doesn't need this classroom. He's graduated.

I sat with that knowledge for the rest of the conference. It didn't make the ache disappear. But it made it bearable.

Real Words *with* Sam

The current American flag has lasted more than 50 years.
Do you think it's time for a new flag?

ONLY IF WE ADD A NEW STATE

If you were to design a new American flag, what would
your flag look like?

I'D MAKE INSTEAD OF STARS, HEARTS

What do you think is the likelihood it's true Betsy Ross
made our flag?

THE STORY IS PROBABLY TRUE

BE HARD TELLING FALSE TALES FOR A
HUNDRED YEARS

Would you want to live in a world that has more or fewer
rules?

I THINK MORE RULES WOULD MAKE THE
WORLD INSTANTLY CRAZY

What do you think about people taking selfies?

A VERY FUN WAY TO CAPTURE MEMORIES

Chapter 24
The 46-Hour Pause

Sam sprang from his chair to retrieve the cue ball—his body suddenly animated in a way I hadn't seen in days.

He wrung his hands. Craned his neck. That familiar jaw-tensing move I've come to recognize: one of his versions of a smile. A flicker of delight, unmistakably his. A signal of engagement.

This was our fourth day onboard the cruise ship, and for the previous forty- six hours. Sam hadn't left our stateroom.

Hours earlier, he'd been a fixture on our balcony, watching the ocean like it held answers to questions I didn't hear. Did his body finally catch up with whatever his mind had been processing out there?

Now we'd been at the sports bar for almost three hours. He'd said he wanted to head back at 7:00. It was past 10:00, and he had no interest in leaving.

We call it The Man Cruise.

It's something Sam and I have done several times now. A father-son trip, simple in structure but big in intention.

I booked this one back in February, and by the time June rolled around, Sam had been counting it down for nearly four months.

He didn't talk about where we were going. Or what we'd do.

Just that we were going.

"Man Cruuuuuise!"

That was enough to make us both smile.

We boarded the ship around 11 a.m. on a Monday. Sam practically bounced his way through the terminal, beaming as he proudly handed his passport to the cruise staff, eager to take the next step.

He kept drifting ahead of me through the roped-off maze of lines, scanning for the right spot like he'd done it a dozen times before. He didn't want to wait for direction. He wanted to lead.

Our stateroom wouldn't be ready for a few hours, so we walked the ship. We visited the muster station, scoped out the theater, checked out the buffet, and found the water slides, which he was most excited about. He'd been talking about them for weeks.

That first meal on board, I had a goal: to help Sam learn how to serve himself at the buffet. He doesn't usually serve himself. Someone else fixes his plate.

But this time, I stood beside him as he worked the tongs, slowly, carefully, to pick up a cheeseburger patty and place it on a bun. It took nearly a full minute. Then fries. Then cookies. And when he sat down to eat, I told him how proud I was. He smiled in that subtle way that tells me he heard it.

After lunch, we found an open perch overlooking the Port of Los Angeles. It was overcast and we stayed there for hours. Sam watched the movement below with calm fascination: buses pulling in, people spilling out with their luggage, cars searching for parking spots. From our rail-side view, he had a clear line of sight to the gangway where passengers were filing onto the ship.

He loves watching motion from above: cars from hotel windows, people moving in patterns. This scene gave him everything he needed. Distance, activity, and time to soak it in.

By the time our stateroom was ready, Sam had no interest in exploring anything else. He went straight to the balcony and stayed there until nightfall. He watched as we pulled away from port, following the small boats trailing alongside, eyes fixed on the slow fade of land behind us. I joined him for a while. We didn't talk much. He didn't move much. But he was at peace. And we were together.

That first day felt like a victory. Sam had navigated new spaces, served himself lunch, and found his rhythm. I was optimistic about the next few days, but with Sam, a win today doesn't promise one tomorrow. Each day starts fresh, with its own set of variables I can't always decode.

The next day proved that point.

In the morning, I thought it might be the right time to head toward the water slide—the one he'd mentioned over 50 times the previous weeks.

But he wouldn't leave the room.

He stayed in bed or sat out on the balcony all day. We didn't eat. He balked at leaving for any reason.

At about 5 p.m., I started the conversation. Pizza. I knew it was a familiar cue. Something he liked. But still: "No." Over and over. Five more minutes. Ten more minutes. Thirty more minutes.

There's no playbook for these moments. Do I wait him out with gentle patience or take a firmer stance? I'm constantly weighing what's loving versus what's just me wimping out.

And all the usual parenting tricks don't work here. Not bribes, not threats, not reverse psychology. Sam would either see right through them or ignore them altogether.

It took more than two hours of gentle negotiation and resetting the clock before he finally agreed to go. It was almost 8 p.m. when he left the room.

We grabbed pizza. Then we wandered over to the sports bar, just across the promenade. We played around on the foosball table for a bit, watching the ball roll, working to hit it with the stick men.

Then he turned his focus to the pool tables. He watched for about 15 minutes, fascinated. When a player scratched, he jumped up and placed the cue ball back on the table, unprompted. People smiled, nodded, and thanked him. He beamed.

After that, I gently steered him into the theater for a show. It was a big production with singing, dancing, and a full stage crew. We sat in the very back row of the balcony. He was anxious. Loud. At the end of the opening number, he clapped vigorously and shouted "Yay!" louder than anyone in the place.

I hoped for at least 30 minutes—he lasted eleven. We left, and I told him how proud I was because he gave it a shot.

I woke up on Wednesday expecting we'd found our rhythm. Maybe yesterday's breakthrough with the theater—even those eleven minutes had been a step forward. Maybe today would bring the water slide he'd been dreaming about.

I was wrong.

———

Just drinking water and breathing ocean air.

He stayed in our stateroom the entire time. Mostly on the balcony, watching the harbor at Catalina or the slow, rhythmic churn of the sea. Every so often, I offered options: a walk, a meal, a show. Even the gym. Anything I could think of.

But every time, the answer was the same:

"No lunch."

"No walk."

"No show."

"The show is closed."

"Maybe next time."

"Sorry, Dad."

Just no.

To everything.

He looked content, and that's what made it harder.

Is he truly at peace—or is he stuck? I never know for sure.

—

Sometimes I'd try to talk with him about plans: the water slide, gym, shows, food. His answers weren't just "no." Sometimes he tossed out times like puzzle pieces.

"11 o'clock!" he'd shout.

"Do you want lunch at 11?"

"No! No 11! One o'clock!"

"What happens at one?"

"No! No one! Six o'clock! Four o'clock!"

He called out the hours like flipping cards from a deck—each one dealt with care, but I didn't know if it was a bluff or a tell.

And with each number came a classic Sam-ism. His own little chorus of comfort and control.

7 o'clock would be followed by *"Seven red tomatoes,"* then a full count: *"One, two, three . . . seven!"*

Another time: *"8 lemons! 2, 4, 6, 8, who do we appreciate? Lemons, lemons, eight lemons!"*

"11 penguins."

"12 eggs."

"10 toes."

Each phrase had its own cadence. Its own history.

These weren't random. They were scripts borrowed from TV, songs, or maybe made up entirely. To him, they're more than repetition. They're rhythm, structure, and self-expression.

To others, it might sound like nonsense.

To me, it's how he makes sense of things.

It's how he wrestles with what his body won't let him do.

Sam doesn't flap his hands much anymore. His self-regulation comes in other forms: pacing, sound effects, scripting—repeating phrases, song lyrics, or numbers with rhythmic precision.

It might sound random to others, but it's not.

These are his tools. His way of helping his body cope when the world asks too much.

And there's one we've found that often helps: taking a deep breath.

If I see him start to tense or tighten, I can say, "Take a breath." And almost always, he does. Big inhale, slow exhale. You can see it in his body—the release, the return.

It helps. But it doesn't fix everything.

And there were moments I wondered if anything would.

I'd nearly given up hope that we'd leave the room before it was time to drive home on Friday.

More than once, I could feel my patience thinning. The balcony was beautiful, sure, but this was our man cruise. And we weren't "doing anything." Every time I gently suggested an idea, Sam got louder. His pushback firm; overwhelming. The more I tried to talk, the more insistent he became.

The man cruise Sam had counted down for four months was slipping away, one refused meal at a time.

I felt frustration. My own body tightening. I knew I had to regulate myself before I pushed him too far.

As we sat on the balcony together, unsure what else to offer, I remembered something.

I spoke out loud—more to myself than to him:

"Okay. I'm taking a breath."

I let him see me do it. Slow in, slow out. Then again.

"I have to remember that this is harder on you than it is on me," I whispered, just loud enough for him to hear.

"As hard as this is for me . . . I know it's harder for you."

I repeated it two, maybe three times.

And something softened. In both of us.

The tension didn't vanish, but it loosened its grip. Time kept slipping. My hope would rise, then fall, then rise again. I could wait again, with patience instead of pressure.

The cycle of numbers and refusals kept coming. The resistance held steady. And then, like a switch, something shifted. Finally, after 46 hours, the pattern changed. I guess that hunger helped his brain get through to his body.

His voice rang out with one of his clearest signals: *"Socks and shoes on!"*

That's his way of saying, "Let's go."

He moved through his ritual like clockwork: shoes, deodorant, teeth, hair. Ready.

He led the way, setting a brisk, focused pace to the buffet. Then he picked up the tongs. Cheeseburger. Fries. Deli meats. Cheese cubes. Grapes.

Focused. Determined.

His fine motor skills made it tough. But he did it—all on his own.

And then…seconds.

Then…*thirds*.

If you know Sam, you know how rare that is. He usually finishes his plate and moves on.

But not this time.

No hesitation, no lingering. He loaded up again.

And I just watched, holding back tears.

I was proud, and I told him so.

—

After dinner, I didn't want to go straight back to the room.

I led him on a longer route. We needed the steps. Ended up at the sports bar again. He gravitated right back to the pool tables. Sat down. Watched. Waited for scratches. Returned cue balls. Friendly, understanding people allowed him to participate.

He was in his element.

Just like two days before: hands wrung, neck craned, jaw clenched. That look I know from trains and roller coasters. It means he's all in.

He'd said he wanted to go back to the room at 7:00. At 10 pm, he showed no sign of wanting to leave the pool table.

I watched the NBA Finals. He watched strangers play pool.

We sat side by side. Regulated. Connected.

From two days of resistance to three hours of pure engagement.

—

This is where I hesitate.

Where I second-guess.

Where I wrestle with whether to push or to wait.

To encourage or to honor stillness.

To nudge forward, or simply be beside him.

That's the line I walk as Sam's dad.

He talked about the water slide every day on the cruise.

He never touched it.

Did he really not want it? Or was it just too hard to begin the movement?

Inertia. And apraxia. A challenging combination to decipher.

I wish I could share Sam's spelled words about what kept him on the balcony for so long and why we never visited the water slide. But we haven't had that conversation yet. For now, I can only witness and wonder.

—

On the last morning, he was joyful. Cooperative. Excited to go home.

And he said it dozens of times:

"I had a great time on the cruise, Dad."

"This was a great cruise."

"We did it!"

Days later, he still says it.

Even with all the no's, resistance, and uncertainty, this was a win.

Not for what we did, but for how we did it. Together.

The best moments weren't loud or flashy. But to us, they shine in the effort, in the trying, in the shared joy of simple things.

Like helping with the cue ball and a deep breath we remembered to take together.

Real Words *with* Sam

What trait do you think you have that shows you are a
good friend?

RESPECT

Give your own synonym for the word powerful?

INFLUENTIAL

What is one way to bring joy to others?

BEING A FRIENDLY COMRADE

Would you find exploration more exciting above the
surface on land or underwater?

DISCOVERING LIFE UNDERWATER BOASTS
MORE POSSIBILITIES

If tomorrow were New Year's Day, what would you resolve?

ID RESOLVE TO RENT OR BUY LANES
AT THE FAIR

What comes to your mind when you think of a puzzle?

DOING HARD PUZZLES TAKES
MENTAL GYMNASTICS

What is one piece of equipment you would want if you
were caught in a flood?

I THINK THAT A CRAFT WOULD
COME IN HANDY

What type of craft?

BOAT

In your own words, tell me about what happened.

A HORRIBLE STORM CAPSIZED A BOAT WITH
EIGHT PASSENGERS ON BOARD

HOWEVER IT WAS BECAUSE OF THE FAMOUS
DUKE THE PEOPLE WERE SAVED

How do you think it felt to be The Duke in this situation?

SURELY IT MUST HAVE BEEN TERRIFYING

Imagine you are part of a rescue mission team, who would you want on your team and why?

BRAD BECAUSE HE IS LEVEL HEADED AND
RESOURCEFUL

HANDY TO HAVE THESE

What is something that you find rewarding?

ALL THE TIMES THAT I ASTOUND
OTHER PEOPLE WITH MY UNEXPECTED
INTELLIGENCE

Chapter 25
Just One Story

This is just one story.

One son.

One family.

One dad still learning how to listen.

Maybe, what you've read here was more than an introduction to Sam.

Maybe it helped you see someone in your life a little differently.

Maybe even yourself.

This book isn't meant to tell the story of autism, or even apraxia.

It's just our window. But I hope it helped you see more clearly through yours.

If you've met one person with autism, you've met one person with autism.

That's true. But I'll add this:

If you've met one person, you've met someone worth knowing—whose intelligence might astound you.

—

In our house, we've learned that seeing isn't believing.

Believing is seeing.

When we start with the assumption that someone has something to say—even when their voice is trapped, even when their body doesn't cooperate, even when the world has written them off—we begin to notice what was always there. Unexpected intelligence, intention behind movement, a person waiting to be known.

It's not a parenting tactic. Or a leadership move.

It's a posture.

A way of living.

A way of seeing.

—

I'll leave you with something Sam spelled when asked: What excites you most about the future?

A CLEAR AND BRIGHT FUTURE LAYS
AHEAD FOR ME

FULL OF ENDLESS ABILITY

Let these be his final words in this book.

But not the end of the conversation.

Because here's what I want to challenge you with:

Read Sam's words again, but this time hear them differently.

Not as inspiration.

As prophecy.

A CLEAR AND BRIGHT FUTURE LAYS
AHEAD FOR ME

FULL OF ENDLESS ABILITY

This isn't just Sam's truth.

It's all of ours—if we're ready to be astounded.

Acknowledgements

Sam, this book is here because of your persistence and your resilience. And, to use your own words, because of your unexpected intelligence. You are my favorite Sam. I love you and I'm proud to be your dad. I am excited to keep learning who you are.

Paulette, there are not enough pages to describe the weight you have carried and the strength you have shown. You've carried us through seasons that demanded far more of you than the rest of us understood. Your love for our family and your steady belief in Sam made space for all of us to grow. This book has my name on it, but your fingerprints are on every chapter. You are the love of my life and I'm blessed to share life with you.

Madison, thank you for being the best daughter I know and the big sister Sam needs. You have walked this path with us from the beginning—loving Sam, protecting him, teasing him, and staying close to him in your own way. You brought light to us in some long years, and I am grateful for the role you play in his life and in ours.

Granny, your presence in our home is an immeasurable blessing. Because you've been here, Paulette and I have had opportunities to show up for each other as husband and wife in ways we never could have managed. Your relationship with Sam is one of the brightest parts of his world. He loves you deeply. Thank you for your steady, seemingly endless patience.

Grant Weber - Even before you joined our family, you made it clear you have Sam's back. As cliché as it sounds, I don't think we could have chosen a better brother-in-law for him.

Our **immediate family** has simply been awesome. You've loved Sam consistently with grace and kindness. Sam talks for months in advance about our December visits to East Bernard, Texas. We know that many people do not have this kind of family support, so we feel exceedingly fortunate.

Thank you to Sam's grandparents, aunts, uncles, and cousins:

Pa and Pal - Thanks for all the extra help and trips to the airport when Sam was very young.

Bob and Laverne, Aunt Suzanne, Uncle Mark, and Bella, Aunt Sandy, Uncle Austin, and Emma, Aunt Christie, Uncle Glenn, with Jordan and Jacob, Uncle Mike, with James and Kathryn, Uncle Steve

and Aunt Loree, with Heather and Hannah, Uncle Craig and Aunt Cindy with Corey, Caitlin, and Carli, Cousin Kendall and Cousin Chris

Sam has been supported by teachers and school staff who showed up for him in classrooms, hallways, and school routines. These are real-life superheroes who deserve far more than a few sentences in the back of this book.

Some had more significant impact than others, but all of you helped write this book through your influence on Sam's learning and development. Thank you to:

Ms. Julia Minderman - You saw ability when others didn't. You were the high school teacher Sam needed to allow him to prove he could do the work.

Mr. Ben Curtain - I was amazed at how you had Sam working with fractions in the 5th grade.

Ms. Kathy Lockridge - Your belief in Sam's potential and encouragement to Paulette was inspiring at a critical time.

Ms. Kimberly Vasquez and **Ms. Rosie Favela** - Your dedication made it possible for Sam to succeed in his Gen Ed academic credit classes.

Mr. K. Krupa - Thanks for being the only Gen Ed teacher to show up to Sam's IEPs and for sharing the ways Sam helped in class and what a joy it was to have him there.

Mr. G. Morse - You believed in Sam's ability when few others did.

Coach J. Drew - Thanks for welcoming Sam into your Gen Ed PE classes.

Mr. Pix, Ms. M. Palmer, Ms. L. Henderson, Mr. G. Cortez, Ms. D. Holemo, Ms. C. Crane, Mr. Cristian, Ms. Ginger, Ms. Wendy, Ms. P. Cline, Ms. J. Hillery, Ms. B Chambliss, Ms. Tara, Ms. L. Helling, Ms. Mary, and so many more aides.

Krista Warren - Thank you for speaking to Sam and all your adult education students as competent adults.

Ms. Gypsy Nieves - You have been a blessing to Sam professionally and personally. Thanks for being his wedding buddy.

Jen Dugas Bitting - Thanks for showing us the path to achieve Sam's high school diploma. Your work grows dignity and respect in a place that matters.

Several professionals outside the school system offered support that reached far beyond academics. These therapists and specialists created environments where Sam could strengthen his skills and explore his abilities. Their work gave our family tools that made a real difference in his daily life.

Thank you to the therapists, specialists, and support providers who played an important role in Sam's growth:

Kasey Howell - Thank you for being a SUPER-STAR in Sam's life. We couldn't adult without you.

Angie Broussard - Your dedication to creating Sam's math curriculum was critical in his early development and thank you for your loving support.

Marcia Boeche - You and the North Coast Church team have been a blessing to Sam and our family. Thank you for your love, patience and Night to Shine.

Gina Mills - Thanks for your positive energy and warm, fun- loving spirit during your many in- home visits.

The ROADS Crew - **Molly McFall and Annie Kesselhaut**

Shauna Jopes and the REINS Therapeutic Horsemanship Program Crew

Briana Hafezi - Sam calls you "MY BRIANA" for a reason. Thank you for being Sam's number one coach, aide, caregiver, and friend—and for caring for him like family. It's not easy for parents to let their child ride away for the day with someone else, but you've made it easy to trust you.

Team Cortica:

Dr. Suzanne Goh - Thanks for creating the Cortica Cares Model and for your wisdom and leadership early in Sam's journey.

Audrey Ketcham - Sam had so much fun with you, especially rock climbing and at the two Night To Shine events you attended with him. We are grateful for how you showed up and honored Sam's dignity, day after day.

Michelle Hardy and Melissa Knopp

Sam communicates through spelling because of people who believed in his intelligence, respected him, and created space for him to be understood.

Thank you to our Spelling Coaches and Communication Partners:

Julie Sando - Working with you started the journey for us. Thank you for your continued support and pioneering leadership in the spelling community.

Dawnmarie Gaivin - You wrote the book on Speller's Method and worked with Sam in ways that helped him progress to sharing original thoughts.

Brooke Poston - Your patience and persistence helped Sam widen his abilities. He expressed an eagerness to get "USED TO OTHER VOICES" and shared how he was excited to get more practice with you.

Ashlyn Isaia - Just wow! The bulk of Sam's deepest and most interesting words have emerged while working with you. Special love and appreciation to you—there's no way this book happens without your skill, consistency, and will. The extra time you invested coaching me and others to be spelling partners for Sam is a priceless gift.

Johnny Perez - We are grateful for your leadership, love of all things motor, and willingness to step in and work with Sam in a pinch.

Thanks to our Fallbrook friends–many of you have shared church life and Bible study groups with us. Others have simply been steady neighbors and friends. You have prayed with us, listened to us, laughed with us, and made sure we never felt alone. Your presence has been an encouragement for our whole family.

Thank you to our local friends:

Jim and Melinda Madden, Brian and Pam Suchoski, Greg and Eva Montague, Jack and Susan O'Connor, Jen Dugas-Bitting and Ken Bitting, Jerry and Adele Maurer, Catie and Chris Timme, Todd and Sandy Goodman, Natalie and Rich Franks, Don and Leanne Green, Alexis Franks, Annie Green, Lindsey Klein, Leah Alford, Greg Hill, Tom and Christy Best with Alexis, Talon, and Augie, Bill and Judy Saunders, Lila Sandshulte, Brad Fox, Heidi and Joe Roderick with Rachelle and Alysha, Phillip and Marti Agassi with Carter, Sherry McFarland, Paige Lawson-Rinehart with Rylee and Dylan, Beth Ann Murray, Banning Cantarini and many others from our Sonrise and North Coast Church Families.

Great neighbors, the Burd, Wise, Heck, and Guinn families.

Sam's friends:
Jakey Braunagel, Cole West, Jacob Clark

We have also been supported by communities that provided connection, resources, and understanding through different seasons of Sam's life.

Thank you to:
Rancho Santa Fe Rotary Club

Paulette's Speller Moms community

TACA (The Autism Community in Action)

Autism One

UA Prayer Warriors

Schlenz Family - Idyllwild Pines Camp

The Autism Society of San Diego

Autism Family Camp (especially cabin 8)

The Autism Legacy Fund

ETSU Lady Lions Volleyball (ET A&M)

Champion Autism - Allison Schnepper

Hope on the Hard Road

Hal Elrod and John Israel - You were the first two people to tell me clearly and directly that this was the book I needed to write. I have begun many books, but it was your encouragement that helped me commit to finish this one.

Thank you, **Hal**.

Thank you, **John**.

Your friendship and guidance helped bring this book into existence. We knew each other long before the world knew your work, and I'm grateful that your voices continue to speak into my life.

This book grew stronger because of people willing to read early pages and offer thoughtful, honest feedback.

Each person who spent time with a draft helped me see something more clearly, tighten a section, or rethink a story. Your insight and encouragement shaped the voice and direction of the book in meaningful ways.

I want to give special recognition to **Bruce and Barbara Goodman**. You read more chapters than anyone else and offered feedback that went far beyond simple encouragement. Your input helped refine key parts of the manuscript, and your belief in the message of this book gave me energy during some important stretches of writing.

Thank you also to everyone who took the time to read a chapter, share impressions, and offer generous feedback along the way:

Ken Morton, Paulette Britton, Madison Britton, Tommy Jean Elliott, Hal Elrod, Jon Berghoff, Pam Suchoski, Rose Fulton, Jeff Bry, Barbara Goodman, Bruce Goodman, Julie Weber, John Kane, Ron Kolb, Krista Warren, Eric Freund, Christen Freund, Sally Chen, Kevin Chen, V John Baker, NJ Yazon, Emma Logan, Kim Koetsier, Lora Pfeifer, Cary Head, Tyler Hudson, Matthew Perry, Laura Poskie, Katrina Hammond, Stacy Barton, Rita Strickland, Joan Dameron, Kasey Howell, Charmaine Tincher, Matt Baker, Laura Sylvester, Johnathan Reeves, Amber Villhaur, Aaron Alba, Don Freda, Kathryn Peraza, Zeena Foteh, Jordan Farber, and Michele Lewis.

Elliot Sylvester - Thank you for learning how to spell and showing me what might be possible for Sam. Watching you spell at the symposium didn't give me certainty, but it cracked the door open enough for us to push forward and see what lay ahead. Your example set us on a path that led to new levels of connection and depth. I am deeply grateful.

This book also came together with the help of professionals who guided the process with skill and steady support.

I want to thank **Amber Vilhauer** and her team at NGNG. Amber's coaching helped me clarify the message I wanted to share, and her team brought consistency and care to the many details of bringing this book to life.

Team NGNG - **Megan O'Malley, Dana Jones, Jess Andrews, Brett Kelly, and Miguel Cordeiro**

The Strong Print Publishing team: **McKenna Reitz and Ashley Bunting**

Ben Williams, Audiobook Engineer, Brand Out Loud Design (BOLD)

To everyone who poured time, energy, and heart into our family and this project, thank you. Your patience, your support, and your willingness to help mean more than you know.

Resources

I've been impacted by dozens of authors, podcasts, online communities, and influencers. Here are a few books I recommend:

Ido in Autismland: Climbing Out of Autism's Silent Prison by Ido Kedar

Best Friends with Autism, Apraxia, and Autonomy: Andrew and Jacob Set Their Voices Free by Jenn Jordan, Andrew Schumacher, and Jakob Jordan

Autism Out Loud: Life with a Child on the Spectrum, from Diagnosis to Young Adulthood by Kate Swenson, Carrie Cariello, and Adrian Wood

Uniquely Human: A Different Way of Seeing Autism by Barry M. Prizant

The Spellers Guidebook: Practical Advice for Parents and Students by Dawnmarie Gaivin, Dana Johnson, and J.B. Handley

For additional reading recommendations and resources, visit: www.RealWordsWithSam.com/resources

About the Authors

J Brad Britton has more than 40 years of experience in sales leadership and organizational development. During his career with Cutco/Vector, he earned eight National Championships and was inducted into the company's Hall of Fame, ranking among the top 15 revenue producers in the company's million-plus-person history.

Today, J Brad works with organizations and leaders, helping them build strong teams, healthy cultures, and meaningful community connections. His work focuses on developing people as much as performance, believing that sustainable success starts with trust and clarity. Whether through business, service, or storytelling, he is committed to helping others bring out the best in those they lead.

For two decades, J Brad assumed his son Sam's limited speech and difficulty following directions reflected limited understanding. In 2018, he watched a non-speaker spell an eloquent sentence and was introduced to spelled communication. That moment opened the door for J Brad and

Sam to begin their own spelling journey, revealing wisdom, humor, and insight that challenged J Brad's beliefs about intelligence and communication.

J Brad lives in Fallbrook, California, with his wife, Paulette, and their family. When he's not working or spelling with Sam, he enjoys live theater, good food, table games, and traveling. *Real Words with Sam* is his first solo book.

Sam Britton is a young man with autism and apraxia whose insights and thoughtful perspective reveal more of who he is each day.

His own phrase, "unexpected intelligence," has shaped this book and continues to influence how his family understands communication, capability, and connection. His contributions to this book reflect his depth, his wit, and his desire to "help others do life."

He loves bowling, watches, computers, music, and spending time with the people he cares about. Sam is also pursuing his high school and college education. He approaches life with enthusiasm, persistence, and a perspective that adds heart and clarity to every chapter.